3 Weeks of Ketogenic Recipes 2021

21 Day Meal Plan + 80 Tasty, Varied & Balanced Recipes That Will Motivate and Help You Get in the Physical Shape You Want

Table of Contents

Introduction

Congratulations on purchasing *3 Weeks of Ketogenic Recipes,* and thank you for doing so. I hope you will find plenty of useful information on the ketogenic diet plan and learn how to use it in your menu planning efficiently. First, let's read a bit about its history.

The Ketogenic methods date back in time. During the progression of history, as early as the 20th century, fasting was theorized by Bernard McFadden, otherwise known as Bernarr Macfadden, as a means for restoring your health. One of his students introduced a treatment for epilepsy using the same plan. In 1912, it was reported by the *New York Medical Journal* that fasting is a successful method to treat epileptic patients, followed by a starch-free and sugar-free diet.

By 1921, Rollin Woodyatt, an endocrinologist, noted the liver produced the ketone bodies (three water-soluble compounds), including acetone, acetoacetate β-hydroxybutyrate, emerging from a diet highly rich in fats and consisting of low amounts of carbohydrates at the same time.

In 1921, Dr. Russell Wilder, who worked for the Mayo Clinic, became well-known when he formulated the ketogenic format, which was then used as part of the epilepsy therapy treatment plan. He had a massive interest in the program because he also had epilepsy. The ketogenic methods also became known for their assistance with weight loss and many other ailments.

As of 2016, Wilder is still functioning successfully without the seizure episodes. It is also noted that the plan is especially recommended for children.

The keto or ketogenic diet is a moderate protein, low-carbohydrate, and higher fat diet technique used to help you effectively burn away body fat. Research and many doctors agree that it will provide you with benefits for your health, weight loss, and overall performance. Go ahead and lose excess body fat without creating those nagging hunger pangs.

The Meaning of Keto

Your body produces ketones, which are small fuel molecules - an alternate fuel source for the body when your blood sugar/glucose is in limited supply.

If you are eating fewer calories and fewer carbs, your liver will produce ketones from the fat that will serve as a fuel source throughout your body - notably your brain. Your brain is a hungry organ that will consume tons of energy daily, and it can't function on fat directly. It can only operate on ketones or glucose. Ketosis is achieved as the body reaches a metabolic state when your body produces these ketones.

Fasting (not eating anything) is the quickest way to achieve ketosis, but you cannot fast indefinitely. The ketogenic diet, on the other hand, allows you to continue in the state of ketosis. The plan holds many of the benefits acquired by fasting, including weight loss, without fasting for the long term.

The Science & Elements of Ketosis: Lipogenesis & Glycogenesis

Two elements that occur when your body doesn't need the glucose:

- *The Stage of Lipogenesis:* If there is a sufficient glycogen supply in your liver and muscles, any excess is converted to fat and stored.

- *The Stage of Glycogenesis:* The excess of glucose converts to glycogen and is stored in the muscles and liver. Research indicates that only about half of your energy used daily can be saved as glycogen.

When the glycerol and fatty acid molecules are released, the ketogenesis process begins, and acetoacetate is produced. The Acetoacetate is converted to two types of ketone units:

- *Acetone:* This is mostly excreted as waste but can also be metabolized into glucose, which is why individuals on a ketogenic diet will experience distinctive smelly breath.

- *Beta-hydroxybutyrate or BHB:* Your muscles will convert the acetoacetate into BHB, which will fuel your brain after you have been on the keto diet for a short time.

Your body will have no more food (similar to when you are sleeping), making your body burn the fat to create ketones. Once the ketones break down the fats, which generate fatty acids, they will burn off in the liver through beta-oxidation.

Thus, when you no longer have a glycogen or glucose supply, ketosis begins and will use the consumed/stored fat as energy.

The meal plan has been calculated using an average of 20 grams daily, but it's up to you to decide your limits. You have plenty of recipes to begin your keto diet.

Let's get started!

Chapter 1: Your Three-Week Meal Plan

You are about to embark on a new way of eating, so be patient with yourself. Follow the meal plan, using leftovers as desired. You can freeze many of the dishes, so enjoy!

Keto uses heavy cream and Italian seasonings in many of its recipes.
If you do not have heavy cream, here is a simple fix for one cup:

- Mix whole milk (.66 or 2/3 cup)
- With melted butter (.33 or 1/3 cup)

It's also very easy to make Italian seasoning.
Combine the following fixings to make three tablespoons of Italian seasoning:

- Dried oregano (1 tbsp.)
- Dried basil (2 tsp.)
- Dried sage (1 tsp.)
- Dried thyme - not ground (2 tsp.)
- Dried rosemary (.5 tsp.)

Week One: Ketogenic Meal Options

Breakfast Time	Lunchtime	Dinnertime	Snack or Dessert
Day One: Best Scrambled Eggs 2.9 g	Buffalo Chicken Soup 4 g	Parmesan Chicken 0.4 g	Cheesecake 3.4 g
Day Two: Macadamia Keto	Snap Pea & Scallion Salad 3 g	Lamb & Asparagus with Tangy Sauce 3.7 g	Leftover Cheesecake 3.4 g

Pancakes 1.5 g			
Day Three: Egg Muffins 1 g	Cauliflower Beef Curry 3 g	Rosemary and Olive Oil Slow Cooked Chicken 1.1 g	Chocolate Roll Cake 3 g
Day Four: Flaxseed Porridge 4 g	Chicken Nuggets 11 g	Broiled Tilapia Parmesan 1.4 g	Leftover Chocolate Roll Cake 3 g
Day Five: Ham & Egg Cups 0.96 g	Cauliflower & Kielbasa Soup 5.7 g	Feta Chicken Burgers 2.5 g	Cheesecake Mocha Bars 3.2 g
Day Six: Baked Custard-Dairy-Free 3 g	Spinach - Broccoli - Feta Salad 4.9 g	Balsamic Grilled Chicken Breast 2.6 g + Cool & Spicy Jicama Slaw 3 g	Leftover Cheesecake Mocha Bars 3.2 g
Day Seven: Sausage Egg Casserole 2.1 g	Smoothie In A Bowl 4 g	Leftover: Balsamic Grilled Chicken Breast 2.6 g + Shortcut Smoky Collard Greens 4 g	Pumpkin Pie Cupcakes 2.9 g

Week Two: Ketogenic Meal Options

I hope you enjoyed the selections for week one. By now, you are starting to see how easy it is to prepare healthy meals without expensive takeout prices!

Breakfast Time	Lunchtime	Dinnertime	Snack or Dessert
Day One: Leftover Pumpkin Pie Cupcakes 2.9 g	Colby Cauliflower Soup & Pancetta Chips 6 g	Shrimp Scampi For Garlic Lovers 1.2 g	Chocolate & Orange Chunk Cookies 2.3 g
Day Two: Cauliflower & Cheddar Hash Browns 2.5 g	Cobb Salad 3 g	Tex-Mex Pork Casserole 8 g	Carrot Cake Fat Bombs 0.9 g
Day Three: Old-Fashioned Baked Custard - Heavy Cream 3 g	Creamy Taco Soup 4 g	Feta Chicken Burgers 2.5 g	Leftover Chocolate & Orange Chunk Cookies 2.3 g
Day Four: Salmon & Cream Cheese Mug Muffin 3 g	Caprese Salad 9 g	Parmesan Chicken 0.4 grams Zucchini Noodle Gratin 3 g	Chocolate Loaf Bread 1.5 g + fresh fruit topping
Day Five: Sausage Egg Casserole	Tuna Salad & Chives 1 g	Chicken & Cheese Stuffed	Leftover Carrot Cake Fat Bombs

		Peppers 5 g	0.9 g
Day Six: Blueberry Flax Microwave Muffin 2.9 g	Leftover Chicken & Cheese Stuffed Peppers 5 g	Crockpot Pork Chops 7.7 + Lavender & Butter Braised Celery 2 g	Leftover Chocolate Loaf Bread 1.5 g + fresh fruit topping
Day Seven: Scrambled Eggs with Mayo 0.99 g	Italian Sausage Soup With Tomatoes & Zucchini Noodles 4 g	Parmesan Shrimp 4.5 g + Mock Potato Casserole 1.6 g	Baked Goat Cheese With Roasted Pistachios & Blackberries 4 g

Week Three: Ketogenic Meal Options

See, I told you that you could do it. If you are at this point in your diet plan, you should be adjusting to the ketogenic menu and its healthy ingredients. Let's begin our three-week journey!

Breakfast Time	Lunchtime	Dinnertime	Snack or Dessert
Day One: Green Smoothie Delight 3 g	Leftover Italian Sausage Soup 4 g	Creamy Chicken Broccoli 5 g	Pumpkin Spice Fat Bombs 0.5 g
Day Two: Bacon & Cheese	BLT Lobster Roll Salad 3 g	Asian Cabbage Stir-Fry 9 g	Gingerbread Spice Dutch Baby

Frittata 2 g			2 g
Day Three: Brunch BLT Wrap 2 g	Chicken Zoodle Soup 4 g	Fiesta Lime Chicken 5.6 g + Bacon-Wrapped Brussel Sprouts 1 g	Leftover Pumpkin Spice Fat Bombs 0.5 g
Day Four: Cinnamon Roll Smoothie 0.6 g	Brunch Cobb Salad Bacon Cups 0.9 g	Sausage Sheet Pan Dinner 7 g	Leftover Gingerbread Spice Dutch Baby 2 g
Day Five: Bagels With Cheese 8 g	Rainbow Salad 1 g	Beef Stroganoff	Coconut- Caramel Bread 3 g
Day Six: Blueberry Muffins 5 g	Leftover Rainbow Salad 1 g	Leftover Fiesta Lime Chicken 5.6 g + Bacon-Wrapped Brussel Sprouts 1 g	Chocolate Sea Salt Cookies 1.6 g
Day Seven: Leftover Blueberry Muffins 5 g	Keto Pizza Chaffles 3 g	Salmon Cakes 3.6 g + Roasted Salt & Pepper Radish Chips 1.2 g	Leftover Chocolate Sea Salt Cookies 1.6 g

Chapter 2: Ketogenic Breakfast Recipes

You will have plenty of breakfast options on the meal plan with a few extras here to substitute or use on your next week of meal planning. Several recipes will call for heavy cream or Italian Seasonings; look in the first chapter for the recipe for these two items. You can make your items from everyday items.

Bacon & Cheese Frittata

Servings Provided: 6
Prep & Cook Time: 45 minutes
Caloric Ratio Measure - Per Serving:
- Kcals: 320
- Net Carbohydrates: 2 g
- Fat Content: 29 g
- Protein: 13 g

Ingredients:
- Heavy cream/see recipe ch.1 (1 cup)
- Eggs (6)
- Crispy slices of bacon (5)
- Chopped green onions (2)
- Cheddar cheese (4 oz./110 g)
- Also Needed: 1 pie plate

Preparation Technique:

1. Warm the oven temperature at 350° Fahrenheit/177° Celsius.
2. Whisk the eggs and seasonings. Empty into the pie pan and top off with the remainder of the fixings. Bake it for 30-35 minutes.
3. Wait for a few minutes before serving for the best results.

Bagels With Cheese

Servings Provided: 6
Prep & Cook Time: 20 minutes
Caloric Ratio Measure - Per Serving:

- Kcals: 374
- Net Carbohydrates: 8 g
- Fat Content: 31 g
- Protein: 19 g

Ingredients:

- Mozzarella cheese (2.5 cups)
- Baking powder (1 tsp.)
- Cream cheese (3 oz./85 g)
- Almond flour (1.5 cups)
- Eggs (2)

Preparation Technique:

1. Shred the mozzarella and combine with the baking powder, flour, and cream cheese in a mixing container. Pop into the microwave for about one minute. Mix well.
2. Let the mixture cool, and add the eggs. Break apart into six sections and shape into round bagels.
3. Note: You can also sprinkle with a seasoning of your choice or pinch of salt if desired.
4. Bake them for approximately 12 to 15 minutes. Serve or cool and store.

Best Scrambled Eggs

Servings Provided: 2
Prep & Cook Time: 10 minutes
Caloric Ratio Measure - Per Serving:
- Kcals: 161.5
- Net Carbohydrates: 2.9 g
- Protein: 13.7 g
- Fat Content: 10.1 g

Ingredients:
- Eggs (4 large)
- Salt and pepper (as desired)
- Skim or 1% milk (.25 cup)
- Fresh parsley (2 tbsp.)
- Cooking oil spray (as needed)

Preparation Technique:

1. Finely chop the parsley. Break eggs into a mixing container with the milk, pepper, salt, and parsley. Whisk until thoroughly combined.
2. Warm a skillet using the med-high temperature setting and lightly spritz it using the cooking spray.
3. Pour eggs into the pan, pushing them around the pan with a non-metal spatula until the eggs are set and no liquid remains (5 min.).
4. Scrape the pan and continue stirring to keep the eggs light and fluffy.
5. Note: For the best results, don't use egg beaters! They will not properly cook.

Brunch BLT Wrap

Servings Provided: 1

Prep & Cook Time: 12-15 minutes

Caloric Ratio Measure - Per Serving:

- Kcals: 256
- Net Carbohydrates: 2 g
- Fat Content: 24 g
- Protein: 8 g

Ingredients:

- Crispy fried bacon slices (4)
- Romaine or Iceberg lettuce leaves (2)
- Chopped tomatoes (.25 cup)
- Mayo (1 tbsp.)
- Optional: Pepper

Preparation Technique:

1. Cook the bacon until crispy in a skillet or the microwave (your choice).
2. Spread a layer of mayonnaise on one side of the lettuce.
3. Add the bacon and tomato. Season the wrap to your liking. Roll it up and serve.

Cauliflower & Cheddar Hash Browns

Servings Provided: 12 hashbrowns
Prep & Cook Time: 30 minutes
Caloric Ratio Measure - Per Serving:

- Kcals: 124
- Net Carbohydrates: 2.5 g
- Protein: 5 g
- Fat Content: 11 g

Ingredients:

- Frozen cauliflower rice - thawed (340 g/12 oz. bag)
- Arrowroot starch (15 g/2 tbsp.)
- Optional: Black pepper, salt, onion powder, garlic powder & other seasonings
- Shredded cheddar cheese (226 g/8 oz. bag)
- Avocado oil (46 g or 1/3 cup)
- Also Needed: Waffle maker

Preparation Technique:

1. Warm a non-stick waffle maker while you prepare the hash brown mixture.
2. Remove most of the liquid from the cauliflower bag by using a knife's tip to poke a tiny hole. Thoroughly squeeze the bag and toss the rice with the seasonings and arrowroot starch in a mixing container.
3. Drizzle in the oil and shredded cheese, tossing to combine.
4. Portion the hash browns into the well's center (leaving the mix piled). Lower the lid to flatten the mixture. Cook until they are a deep golden brown. When done, the cheese will be crispy, making it easy to pop out of the waffle iron.

Alternative Cooking Methods:

5. Option 1: You can also use a generously greased muffin tin in a 475° Fahrenheit/246° Celsius oven until crispy on the outside edges (10 min.).

6. Option 2: Prepare a non-stick skillet using the med-high temperature setting. Shape the portions into thick patties and fry on each side until crispy and golden brown.

Egg Muffins

Servings Provided: 12
Prep & Cook Time: 35 minutes
Caloric Ratio Measure - Per Serving:
- Kcals: 147
- Net Carbohydrates: 1 g
- Fat Content: 11 g
- Protein: 10 g

Ingredients:
- Eggs (12)
- Italian sausage (.5 lb./230 g)
- 36% heavy cream (.25 cup)
- Garlic powder (.5 tsp.)
- Chives (2 tsp.)
- Himalayan pink salt (1-2 pinches)
- Also Needed: 12-count muffin tin

Preparation Technique:

1. Warm the oven to reach 350° Fahrenheit/177° Celsius.
2. Brown the sausage until thoroughly browned and cooked. Cool the meat in the pan, but do *not* drain off the fat.
3. Break the eggs into a large mixing container and add the cream. Mix and thoroughly whisk in the seasonings and any optional add-ins.
4. Fold in the meat and thoroughly mix it. Scoop it into a dozen well-greased muffin wells.
5. Bake for ½ hour or until the egg centers are set.

Ham & Egg Cups

Servings Provided: 9

Prep & Cook Time: 25 minutes

Caloric Ratio Measure - Per Serving:
- Kcals: 117
- Net Carbohydrates: 0.96 g
- Protein: 7.72 g
- Fat Content: 9.17 g

Ingredients:
- Fresh eggs, fresh (5 large/250 g)
- 36% heavy cream/see recipe ch.1 (.5 cup/135 g)
- Natural-Uncured Black Forest Ham (7 oz./200 g pkg.)
- Coconut oil (5 grams/1 tsp.)
- Also Needed: Muffin tin (at least 9-count)

Preparation Technique:

1. Set the oven temperature at 425° Fahrenheit/218° Celsius.
2. Lightly grease nine wells/cups of a muffin tin with a spritz of cooking oil.
3. Arrange one slice of ham in each of the muffin wells/cups, pressing the ham's slices into the cups centered with the ham covering the sides and bottoms.
4. Whisk and thoroughly combine the cream, egg, pepper, and salt.
5. Fill nine of the muffin cups.
6. Bake until the egg centers have puffed, and the eggs are entirely set (7-10 min). They might slightly jiggle - if shaken but shouldn't be runny/liquidy.
7. Add desired garnishes such a green onion or roasted red peppers or feta cheese, but add the extra carbs.

Macadamia Keto Pancakes

Servings Provided: 4

Prep & Cook Time: 20 minutes

Caloric Ratio Measure - Per Serving:
- Kcals: 300
- Net Carbohydrates: 1.5 g
- Fat Content: 30 g
- Protein: 6 g

Ingredients:
- Macadamia nuts – roasted (30 g/1.1 oz)
- Raw egg (28 g/1 oz.)
- Optional: Vanilla extract (3 drops)
- Pecan/macadamia nut oil (6 g/0.2 oz.)

Preparation Technique:

1. Finely chop the nuts in a blender.
2. Thoroughly whisk the egg, add it to the oil, and into the nuts.
3. Add vanilla if desired.
4. Lightly spritz a skillet using a baking oil spray.
5. Drop the batter into desired size circles and cook until nicely browned to serve.

Salmon & Cream Cheese Mug Muffin

Servings Provided: 2

Prep & Cook Time: 10 minutes

Caloric Ratio Measure - Per Serving:

- Kcals: 374
- Net Carbohydrates: 3 g
- Fat Content: 32 g
- Protein: 17 g

Ingredients:

The Mug Muffin Mix:

- Flax meal (.25 cup)
- Almond flour (.25 cup)
- Baking soda (.25 tsp.)
- Water (2 tbsp.)
- Coconut milk/cream (2 tbsp.)
- Organic/free-range egg (1 large)
- Salt (1 pinch)

- Smoked salmon
- Spring onion/chives (2 tbsp.)
- Sour cream/full-fat cream cheese (2 portions)

Preparation Technique:

1. Combine all of the dry components, and blend in the water, cream, and egg. Mix well with a fork.
2. Finely chop the chives and slice the salmon. Add to the mixture.
3. Microwave for 60 to 90 seconds on high.
4. Add the garnishes and enjoy.

**You can also bake at 350° Fahrenheit/177° Celsius for 12 to 15 minutes (for 4 to 8 servings) if you don't have a microwave.

Sausage Egg Casserole

Servings Provided: 12
Prep & Cook Time: 30 minutes
Caloric Ratio Measure - Per Serving:
- Kcals: 200.5
- Net Carbohydrates: 2.1 g
- Protein: 15.7 g
- Fat Content: 39.4 g

Ingredients:
- Cooked - browned breakfast sausage - low-fat & reduced-sodium (12 oz./340 g)
- Eggs (12 large)
- Skim milk (.25 cup)
- Low-fat cheddar cheese (2 cups - shredded)
- Black pepper (.25 tsp.)

Preparation Technique:

1. Set the oven to 375° Fahrenheit/191° Celsius.
2. Use paper or lightly grease a 12-count muffin pan or grease a casserole dish.
3. Add the batter and bake for ½ hour. Cool for five minutes before serving.

Scrambled Eggs with Mayo

Servings Provided: 1
Prep & Cook Time: 15 minutes
Caloric Ratio Measure - Per Serving:
- Kcals: 307
- Net Carbohydrates: 0.99 g
- Protein: 6.6 g
- Fat Content: 30.81 g

Ingredients:
- Large raw egg (1 @ 1.8 oz. or 50 g)
- Butter (0.4 oz. or 10 g)
- Organic mayonnaise (0.8 oz. or 23 g)
- Salt (1 pinch)

Preparation Technique:

1. Prepare a small pan to melt the butter.
2. Whisk the mayo with the egg until thoroughly mixed.
3. Cook and swirl the egg until done. Serve promptly.

Breakfast Porridge Cereal

Flaxseed Porridge

Servings Provided: 1

Prep & Cook Time: 5 minutes

Caloric Ratio Measure - Per Serving:
- Net Carbohydrates: 4 g
- Protein: 6 g
- Fat Content: 40 g

Ingredients:
- Flaxseed - plain or roasted is nutty-like (3 tbsp.)
- Coconut milk - unsweetened (.5 cup)
- Butter (2.5 tsp.)
- Grapeseed oil (2 tsp.)
- Wild/frozen blueberries (2 tbsp.)
- Cinnamon (0.125 tsp.)

Preparation Technique:

1. Whisk the milk with the flaxseed in a microwave-safe bowl. Use one that will hold at least two cups of liquid. Cook until the mixture starts rising (30-45 sec.).
2. Transfer the container to the countertop and wait for it to cool for one minute.
3. Mix in the butter, oil, blueberries, and cinnamon. Stir thoroughly to coat the blueberries. Don't over-stir; it will make the porridge gummy.
4. *Note:* You can also make it using a small saucepan on the stovetop. Combine the fixings provided and transfer the pan from the heated burner once it begins boiling.

Breakfast Custard Options

Baked Custard - Dairy-Free

Servings Provided: 6

Prep & Cook Time: 1 hour 20 minutes

Caloric Ratio Measure - Per Serving:
- Kcals: 246
- Net Carbohydrates: 3 g
- Protein: 6 g
- Fat Content: 24 g

Ingredients:
- Unsweetened - full-fat coconut milk (3 cups/678 g)
- Raw eggs (4 large/200 g)
- Pure vanilla extract (1 tsp./2.5 g) or scrapings from ½ of a vanilla pod
- Optional Sprinkle Topping: Nutmeg/cinnamon
  Also Needed:
- Glass baking dish - to hold serving containers
- Glass custard/serving dishes (6 oz./170 g)

Preparation Technique:

1. Warm the oven to 350° Fahrenheit/177° Celsius.
2. Boil enough water to come ½-inch from the top of the outside of the custard cups. Place the cups into the pan. (Wait to fill the dish with water.)
3. Whisk the eggs with the milk, sweetener, and vanilla and add them to the cups. Sprinkle cinnamon/nutmeg over the top as desired.
4. Arrange the holding tray on the oven rack and pour the hot water to make the water bath. Bake the custard for 45 minutes.
5. Check for doneness. Insert a knife into the middle of the cup. It's ready if the knife is clean.
6. Carefully transfer the dishes to the countertop or serving tray to serve. Add any leftovers to the fridge with a covering of foil or plastic wrap.

Old-Fashioned Baked Custard - Heavy Cream

Servings Provided: 6

Prep & Cook Time: 1 hour 20 minutes

Caloric Ratio Measure - Per Serving:

- Kcals: 370
- Net Carbohydrates: 3 g
- Protein: 6 g
- Fat Content: 37 g

Ingredients:

- Water (.5 cup)
- 36% heavy cream/see recipe ch.1 (2.5 cups/565 g)
- Raw egg (4 large/200 g)
- Pure vanilla extract (1 tsp./2.5 g) or Pod scrapings (½ of a vanilla pod)
  Optional Toppings:
- Sweetener - your preference
- Nutmeg or cinnamon

- Glass baking dish
- Glass custard dishes (6 oz./170 g)

Preparation Technique:

1. Measure and boil water to make a water bath using the baking dish. It needs to be enough to extend three-quarters of the way up the custard cups (fill in the last step).
2. Set the oven at 350° Fahrenheit/177° Celsius.
3. Use a mixing container to whisk the eggs with the water, vanilla, cream, and sweetener - if using.
4. Scoop the custard into the serving cups. (Place the cups in the baking dish before you begin.) Sprinkle using a dusting of the nutmeg or cinnamon to your liking.
5. Arrange the baking dish on the oven rack. Pour the hot water into the ½-inch marker of the cups.
6. Set a timer to bake for 45 minutes. It should be firmly set. Test it using a knife in the centermost part of the custard. If it's removed and it's "custard-free," the custard is ready to be served.
7. Enjoy the warm dish of custard or store it with a covering of foil

or plastic in the refrigerator.

Muffins

Blueberry Flax Microwave Muffin

Servings Provided: 1
Prep & Cook Time: 2 minutes
Caloric Ratio Measure - Per Serving:
- Kcals: 160.1
- Net Carbohydrates: 2.9 g
- Protein: 9.2 g
- Fat Content: 9.6 g

Ingredients:
- Frozen blueberries (1 oz./28 g)
- Ground flaxseed (.25 cup)
- Baking powder (.5 tsp.)
- Pancake syrup - sugar-free (2 tbsp.)
- Egg (1 white)
- Orange zest (.5 tsp.)
- Nutmeg (.5 tsp.)
- Also Needed: Organic coconut oil spray
- Optional: Butter & pancake syrup

Preparation Technique:

1. Thoroughly whisk the dry fixings (preferably in a large measuring cup) and add the rest of the fixings with the flax - add the egg, zest, and syrup.
2. Pour the mixture into an oversized coffee cup sprayed with the oil. Pop it in the microwave for a tall muffin (1.5 min.).
3. Note: Use a shallow cereal container or ramekin for a flat muffin top.
4. Top with a portion of butter and syrup as desired - but count the carbs.

Blueberry Muffins

Servings Provided: 12

Prep & Cook Time: 55 minutes

Caloric Ratio Measure - Per Serving:
- Kcals: 221
- Net Carbohydrates: 5 g
- Protein: 6 g
- Fat Content: 20 g

Ingredients:
- Almond flour (2 cups/224 g)
- Coconut flour (.25 cup/30 g)
- Konjac root fiber (2 tsp./8 g)
- Baking powder & soda (4 g/1 tsp. each)
- Salt (1 pinch)
- Olive oil (.5 cup/108 g)
- Fresh eggs (3 large/150 g)
- Water (2-4 tbsp.)
- Fresh blueberries (.5 cup/74 g)

Preparation Technique:

1. Set the oven temperature at 350° Fahrenheit/177° Celsius.
2. Cover the muffin tin with 12 paper/foil liners.
3. Whisk/sift the almond flour with the baking soda and powder, konjac root fiber, salt, and coconut flour.
4. Mix in the eggs with olive oil and two tablespoons of water into the dry components. Thoroughly whisk to combine (as the consistency of thick pancake batter).
5. Gently fold in the blueberries (about half to two-thirds full).
6. Bake the muffins till done (35-40 min.), testing them using a toothpick. Push it into the middle of the muffin. When removed, it should be clean if it's done.
7. Serve warm or chilled.

Delicious Ketogenic Bread Options

If you have concerns and are not sure of whether you can use bread and remain on keto; put those worries away and enjoy one of these:

Cheddar Bread

Servings Provided: 1
Prep & Cook Time: 5 minutes
Caloric Ratio Measure - Per Serving:
- Kcals: 289.2
- Net Carbohydrates: 1.4 g
- Fat Content: 22.5 g
- Protein: 16.4 g

Ingredients:
- Egg (1 large)
- Flaxseed meal (2 tbsp.)
- Baking powder (.5 tsp.)
- Swerve sweetener (a pinch/as desired)
- Cheddar cheese - shredded (.25 cup)
- Butter - melted (1 tsp.)

Preparation Technique:

1. Melt the butter in a flat container or 430 g/15 oz. - oval ramekin.
2. Whisk and add in the egg, baking powder, flax meal, and sweetener of choice.
3. Add the cheddar cheese and mix and pop it into the microwave for one minute.
4. Flip the bread oven and microwave it for another ten seconds - if it's not done in the middle of 1 slice of bread.
5. Slice it in half and top it with the desired sandwich filling.
6. Note: Add a pinch of parsley to the mix for a change of pace.

Flatbread

Servings Provided: 1

Prep & Cook Time: 55 minutes

Caloric Ratio Measure - Per Serving:
- Net Carbohydrates: 4 g
- Protein: 27 g
- Fat Content: 39 g

Ingredients:
- Mozzarella cheese - part-skim - shredded (.75 cup or 75 g)
- Egg (1 large/50 g)
- Unchilled cream cheese - Philadelphia brand (1.5 tbsp./35 g)
- Olive oil (1 tbsp./10 g)
- Coconut flour - ex. - Bob's Red Mill (1 tsp./2.5 g)

- Black pepper
- Garlic powder
- Salt
- Xanthan gum (0.1 g)

Preparation Technique:

1. Set the oven temperature at 350° Fahrenheit/177° Celsius.
2. Prepare a baking tray with a layer of parchment baking paper.
3. Combine the egg and cream cheese using a fork until thoroughly combined.
4. Mix in the rest of the fixings and spread it over the pan in an eight-inch circle.
5. Bake for about ½ hour on the centermost oven rack.
6. Flip the flatbread over during the last ten minutes of cooking.

Flax Bread

Servings Provided: 8 - varies **Prep
& Cook Time**: 20 minutes **Caloric
Ratio Measure - Per Serving**:

- Net Carbohydrates: 6 g
- Protein: 14 g
- Fat Content: 42 g

Ingredients:

- Almond meal (almond flour (1.2 oz./35 g)
- Flaxseed meal (whole ground flaxseed (1.4 oz./40 g)
- Baking powder (0.1 oz./4 g)
- Salt (o.1 oz./1.5 g)
- Vinegar - white distilled (any brand (0.1 oz./2 g)
- Liquid stevia (4 drops)
- Raw mixed egg (3 oz./85 g)
- Melted - coconut oil (1.1 ounces/31 g) or butter (1.3 ounces/37 g)
- Also Needed: 8 x 8-inch/20x20-cm pan

Preparation Technique:

1. Heat the oven at 350° Fahrenheit/177° Celsius.
2. Weigh all ingredients and combine the dry ones - first. Then mix in the wet ones.
3. Lightly grease the baking pan and add the bread.
4. Bake for eight to ten minutes. Slice with a knife and lift it from the pan with a spatula.

High-Fiber Keto Flax Rolls

Servings Provided: 4
Prep & Cook Time: 45 minutes
Caloric Ratio Measure - Per Serving:

- Kcals: 113
- Net Carbohydrates: 0.7 g
- Fat Content: 10.65 g
- Protein: 2.3 g

Ingredients:

- Flax meal (0.5 oz./13 g)
- Salt (1 pinch)
- Whole psyllium husks (.4 oz./12 g)
- Baking powder & soda (1 g each)
- Raw egg (1.8 oz./50 g)
- Oil - keto-friendly choice (1.2 oz./35 g)
- Cider vinegar (0.1 oz./4 g)

Preparation Technique:

1. Warm the oven temperature at 300° Fahrenheit/149° Celsius.
2. Prepare a baking tray with a layer of parchment baking paper.
3. Whisk the egg, oil, water, and vinegar. Mix in the baking soda, flax meal, baking powder, psyllium husks, and salt. Thoroughly combine the fixings.
4. Wait for about five minutes for the dough to "rest."
5. Portion the prepared dough into four rolls. You can weigh if desired.
6. Dampen your hands and shape the dough as desired. Place them on the baking tray.
7. Set the oven timer to bake for ½ hour.

Chapter 3: Ketogenic Lunchtime Recipes

About mid-day, you will probably feel a bit hungry. Why not enjoy a dish of salad or bowl of soup?

Brunch Cobb Salad Bacon Cups

Servings Provided: 6

Prep & Cook Time: 1 hour 5 minutes

Caloric Ratio Measure - Per Serving:

- Kcals: 145
- Net Carbohydrates: 0.9 g
- Fat Content: 9.9 g
- Protein: 9.5 g

Ingredients:

- Thin-cut bacon (12 slices)
- Romaine lettuce (1 cup)
- Cooked chicken (.5 cup)
- California Avocado (half of 1)
- Hard-boiled egg (1)
- Tomato (.25 cup)

- Bleu cheese (2 tbsp.)
- Dressing of choice

Preparation Technique:

1. Finely chop the lettuce and slice the egg. Chop the chicken, tomato, and avocado. Crumble the cheese and set it aside.
2. Set the oven at 425° Fahrenheit/218° Celsius.
3. Cover the wells of a standard-sized muffin tin using a sheet of foil.
4. Slice six of the bacon slices in half and cover each cup with two halves - forming an x-type pattern (using the whole piece and secure it with a toothpick).
5. Bake them for about 35 minutes until the bacon is crunchy, and cool them for about 20 minutes. Remove the toothpicks and fill

the cups.

6. Top it off with your favorite dressing (or not) and serve.

Soup

Buffalo Chicken Soup

Servings Provided: 6

Prep & Cook Time: 40 minutes

Caloric Ratio Measure - Per Serving:
- Kcals: 335
- Net Carbohydrates: 4 g
- Protein: 33 g
- Fat Content: 17 g

Ingredients:
- Olive oil (1 tbsp.)
- Onion (1 medium)
- Garlic powder (1 tsp.)
- Chopped celery (2 cups)
- Dried thyme (1 tsp.)
- Chicken breasts (4)
- Hot sauce (.25 cup/as desired)
- Chicken stock (4 cups)
- Cream cheese (4 oz./110 g)
- Blue cheese - crumbled (.5 cup + more to serve)

Preparation Technique:

1. Dice the celery and onion.

2. Set the Instant Pot using the sauté mode to warm the oil. Dice/chop and add the celery and onions. Sauté them until they're starting to soften.

3. Measure and shake in the garlic powder and thyme. Sauté the mixture for a couple of minutes.

4. Meanwhile, trim the chicken and remove the skin and bones. Slice it into lengthwise strips.

5. Toss the chicken, hot sauce, and chicken stock into the cooker.

6. Securely close the lid and set the timer for 15 minutes using the

high-pressure setting.

7. At that time, natural-release the pressure for ten minutes. Next, quick-release the remainder of the built-up steam.

8. Dice the cream cheese into chunks and crumble the blue cheese.

9. Transfer the chicken to a cutting block to dice/shred it into chunks.

10. Next, mix in both varieties of cheese to the hot soup and wait for it to melt while you're shredding the chicken.

11. Whisk the soup and add the shredded chicken back into the pot.

12. Serve it hot with the blue cheese and hot sauce to your liking.

Cauliflower Beef Curry

Servings Provided: 4

Prep & Cook Time: 30 minutes

Caloric Ratio Measure - Per Serving:

- Kcals: 518
- Net Carbohydrates: 3 g
- Fat Content: 34.6 g
- Protein: 44.6 g

Ingredients:

- Cauliflower florets (1 head)
- Ground beef (1.5 lb./680 g)
- Olive oil (2 tbsp.)
- Allspice (.25 tsp.)
- Cumin (.5 tsp.)
- Garlic-ginger paste (1 tbsp.)
- Whole tomatoes (6 oz./170 g can)
- Chili pepper & salt (to your liking)
- Water (.25 cup)

Preparation Technique:

1. Warm a skillet using the medium-temperature setting. Pour in the oil and the beef to cook for five minutes.
2. Stir in the tomatoes, cauliflower allspice, salt, chili pepper, and cumin. Sauté it for six minutes.
3. Pour in the water and wait for it to boil ten minutes or until the liquids have reduced by about half.
4. Serve it warm.

Cauliflower & Kielbasa Soup

Servings Provided: 4

Prep & Cook Time: 40 minutes

Caloric Ratio Measure - Per Serving:
- Kcals: 251
- Net Carbohydrates: 5.7 g
- Protein: 10 g
- Fat Content: 19 g

Ingredients:
- Ghee (3 tbsp.)
- Cauliflower (1 head)
- Rutabaga (1)
- Kielbasa sausage (1)
- Chicken broth (2 cups)
- Small onion (1)
- Water (2 cups)
- Black pepper and salt (as desired)

Preparation Technique:

1. Chop the cauliflower, onions, and rutabaga. Slice the sausage.
2. Melt two tablespoons of the ghee in a soup pot. Sauté it for three minutes.
3. Toss in the rutabaga and cauliflower. Sauté it for about five minutes.
4. Add the broth, water, salt, and pepper. Boil for about 20 minutes.
5. Prepare a skillet, add the butter, and fry the sausage (5 min.).
6. Puree the soup until it's smooth and serve with the kielbasa.

Chicken 'Zoodle' Soup

Servings Provided: 2
Prep & Cook Time: 15 minutes
Caloric Ratio Measure - Per Serving:
- Kcals: 310
- Net Carbohydrates: 4 g
- Fat Content: 16 g
- Protein: 34 g

Ingredients:
- Chicken breast (1)
- Zucchini (1)
- Avocado oil (2 tbsp.)
- Chicken broth (3 cups)
- Green onion (1)
- Celery stalk (1)
- Cilantro (.25 cup)
- Salt (to your liking)

Preparation Technique:

1. Chop or dice the breast of the chicken. Peel the zucchini.
2. Add the oil to a saucepan. Cook the chicken until done. Pour in the broth and simmer.
3. Chop the celery and green onions and toss them into the pan. Simmer for three to four more minutes.
4. Chop the cilantro and prepare the zucchini noodles. Use a potato peeler or spiralizer to make the 'noodles.' Add to the pot.
5. Cook for several more minutes and season as desired.

Colby Cauliflower Soup & Pancetta Chips

Servings Provided: 4

Prep & Cook Time: 30 minutes

Caloric Ratio Measure - Per Serving:

- Kcals: 402
- Net Carbohydrates: 6 g
- Protein: 8 g
- Fat Content: 37 g

Ingredients

- Cauliflower florets (2 heads)
- Onion (1)
- Ghee (2 tbsp.)
- Water (2 cups)
- Almond milk (3 cups)
- Shredded Colby cheese (1 cup)
- Pancetta strips (3)

Preparation Technique:

1. Chop the cauliflower and onion. Shred the cheese.
2. Prepare a saucepan and melt the butter. Toss in the onion to sauté for three minutes. Mix in the cauliflower and sauté for three more minutes.
3. Add the pepper, salt, and water - wait for it to boil. Lower the temperature setting to simmer for ten minutes.
4. Puree the cauliflower and stir in the milk and cheese. When it's melted, adjust the seasonings to your liking.
5. Prepare the pancetta until crispy in a skillet. Toss it over the soup and serve.

Creamy Taco Soup

Servings Provided: 4

Prep & Cook Time: 45 minutes

Caloric Ratio Measure - Per Serving:
- Kcals: 347
- Net Carbohydrates: 4 g
- Protein: 21 g
- Fat Content: 27 g

Ingredients:
- Ground chicken/turkey/beef (1 lb./450 g)
- Olive/other cooking oil (1 tbsp.)
- Small onion (1)
- Cloves of garlic (2-3)
- Optional: Green bell pepper (1 small)
- Rotel tomatoes (10 oz./280 g can) or Large tomato (1)
- Cream cheese (230 g/8 oz. pkg.) or (Heavy cream (1 cup)
- Taco seasoning (1 pkg.) homemade ok (2 tbsp.)
- Salt & pepper (as desired)
- Beef broth (14.5 oz. can/1.5 cups)

Preparation Technique:

1. Add one tablespoon of oil to a large pot. Brown the beef, garlic, and onion using the med-high temperature setting for seven to eight minutes or until the ground beef is browned thoroughly.
2. Dice the garlic, onion, pepper, and tomatoes.
3. Mix in the bell pepper, cream cheese, tomatoes, and spices. Stir the mixture for four to five minutes or until the tomatoes are softened, and cream cheese is mixed.
4. Dump the beef broth into the soup mixture and lower the heat setting to the med-low function. Simmer it until the desired thickness is achieved (15-20 min.).
5. Serve it using freshly sliced avocado, jalapenos, sour cream, freshly minced cilantro, shredded cheese, and a drizzle of lime.

Italian Sausage Soup With Tomatoes & Zucchini Noodles

Servings Provided: 8

Prep & Cook Time: varies - 2 hours

Caloric Ratio Measure - Per Serving:
- Kcals: 497
- Net Carbohydrates: 4 g
- Protein: 55 g
- Fat Content: 27 g

Ingredients:
- Turkey/pork Italian sausage (19.5 oz./550 g pkg.)
- Olive oil (1 tbsp.)
- Chicken stock (8 cups/1.9-L. - from a carton/can/homemade)
- Tomato paste (2 tbsp.)
- Petite tomatoes - diced (2 cans/14.5 oz./410 g each)
- Dried basil (1 tbsp.)
- Dried Greek oregano (2 tsp.)
- Optional: Ground fennel (2 tsp.)
- Green & red bell peppers (half of each one)
- Onion (half of one medium)
- Medium zucchini (2 @10-inches/25-cm long)
- Black pepper & salt (as desired)

Preparation Technique:

1. Chop the onions and peppers.

2. Heat a skillet with a bit of oil and add the sausage to cook until it's browned thoroughly.

3. Combine the sausage, tomato paste, diced tomatoes, chicken stock, and spices into the soup pot. Wait for it to simmer.

4. Dice the bell peppers and onion. Sauté them for a few minutes and toss them into the soup. Simmer them using the low-temperature setting (30-60 min.).

5. Prepare the zucchini into noodles using a veggie peeler or spiralizer. Add them to the soup and simmer on low (20-30 min.).

6. Serve them hot, with a portion of freshly grated parmesan as desired.

Salad

BLT Lobster Roll Salad

Servings Provided: 4

Prep & Cook Time: 8-10 minutes**

Caloric Ratio Measure - Per Serving:
- Kcals: 3
- Net Carbohydrates: 3 g
- Fat Content: 28 g
- Protein: 19 g

Ingredients:

The Salad:
- Cauliflower florets - cooked (1.5 cups)
- Lobster meat (2 cups)
- Sugar-free mayonnaise (.5 cup)
- Fresh tarragon leaves (1 tsp.)

- Romaine lettuce (8 leaves)
- Cooked bacon (.5 cup)
- Tomatoes (.5 cup)

Preparation Technique:

1. Chop the meat from the lobster.
2. Cook the bacon. Chop the bacon, tarragon, and tomatoes.
3. Mix the cauliflower, lobster, tarragon, and mayonnaise in a container and mix until creamy.
4. Place the leaves of lettuce in a serving container. Add the prepared mixture evenly.
5. Sprinkle with the garnishes and serve chilled or room temperature.
6. Note: Times do not count cooking the cauliflower or bacon.

Healthy Cobb Salad

Servings Provided: 2

Prep & Cook Time: 10 minutes

Caloric Ratio Measure - Per Serving:

- Kcals: 600 g
- Net Carbohydrates: 3 g
- Fat Content: 48 g
- Protein: 43 g

Ingredients:

- Hard-boiled egg (1)
- Spinach (1 cup)
- Bacon (2 strips)
- Campari tomato (half of 1)
- Chicken breast (2 oz./56 g)
- Avocado (¼ of 1)
- Olive oil (1 tbsp.)
- White vinegar (.5 tsp.)

Preparation Technique:

1. Prepare the chicken and bacon and shred/slice the chicken – your choice.
2. _Cut all of the ingredients into bits._
3. _Toss the salad in a mixing container and mix with oil and vinegar._
4. Toss gently to serve.

Keto Caprese Salad

Servings Provided: 2

Prep & Cook Time: 6-8 minutes

Caloric Ratio Measure - Per Serving:

- Kcals: 189 g
- Net Carbohydrates: 9 g
- Fat Content: 12 g
- Protein: 9 g

Ingredients:

- Fresh mozzarella (.5 lb. or 230 g)
- Tomato (1 large)
- Balsamic reduction (1 tbsp.)
- Olive oil (1 tbsp.)
- Basil (4 leaves)
- Pepper and salt (1 pinch each)

Preparation Technique:

1. Slice/dice the cheese and the tomatoes. Intertwine them in the serving dish.
2. Drizzle with the oil and balsamic reduction.
3. Garnish as desired.

Rainbow Salad

Servings Provided: 8

Prep & Cook Time: 6-7 minutes

Caloric Ratio Measure - Per Serving:
- Kcals: 109 g
- Net Carbohydrates: 1 g
- Fat Content: 9 g
- Protein: 15 g

Ingredients:

The Dressing:
- Garlic cloves (2)
- Parsley (.25 cup)
- White balsamic vinegar (.5 cup)
- Olive oil (2 tbsp.)
- Salt & pepper (1 pinch)

- Red cabbage (2 cups)
- Assorted salad greens (8 cups)
- Carrots (1 cup)
- Cucumber (1 cup)
- Raw sunflower seeds (.5 cup)
- Red & yellow bell pepper (1 each)

Preparation Technique:

1. Do the prep and measure all the fixings.
2. Mince the garlic and parsley. Chop the peppers, cabbage, and cucumber. Slice the carrots.
3. Whisk all of the dressing fixings in a mixing container. Pour into a serving container.
4. Drain the chickpeas and prep the veggies.
5. Prepare the salads and serve.

Snap Pea & Scallion Salad - Hot

Servings Provided: 1

Prep & Cook Time: 10 minutes + chill time

Caloric Ratio Measure - Per Serving:
- Net Carbohydrates: 3 g
- Protein: 2 g
- Fat Content: 14 g

Ingredients:
- Sugar snap peas (1.8 oz./50 g)
- Scallions - green & white parts (0.4 oz./10 g)
- Sesame oil (0.1 oz./2 g)
- Coconut aminos/or another keto-friendly soy sauce (2 g/.1 oz)
- Cider vinegar (0.1 oz./3 g)
- Olive oil (0.4 oz./11 g)
- Garlic powder (0.1 g)
- Sesame seeds (0.1 oz./2 g)
- Optional Ingredient: Red chili flakes

Preparation Technique:

1. Slice the snap peas and diagonally slice the scallions.
2. Combine the sliced veggies with the rest of the fixings, tossing thoroughly.
3. Use a plastic wrap sheet to cover the container - pop it into the fridge for at least two hours.
4. Serve with your favorite meat choice.

Spinach - Broccoli - Feta Salad

Servings Provided: 4

Prep & Cook Time: 15 minutes

Caloric Ratio Measure - Per Serving:

- Kcals: 397
- Net Carbohydrates: 4.9 g
- Fat Content: 3.8 g
- Protein: 9 g

Ingredients:

- Vinegar - white wine (1 tbsp.)
- Olive oil (2 tbsp.)
- Broccoli slaw (2 cups)
- Poppy seeds (2 tbsp.)
- Spinach (2 cups)
- Black pepper & salt (as desired)
- Walnuts (.33 cup)
- Sunflower seeds (.33 cup)
- Blueberries (.33 cup)
- Feta cheese (.66 cup crumbled)

Preparation Technique:

1. Chop the spinach and nuts.
2. Combine the slaw, spinach, blueberries, sunflower seeds, walnuts, and cheese.
3. Make the dressing (vinegar, oil, salt, pepper, and poppy seeds) and add to the salad.
4. Toss it and serve.

Chapter 4: Ketogenic Dinnertime Recipes

Seafood & Fish

Broiled Tilapia Parmesan

Servings Provided: 2

Prep & Cook Time: 15 minutes

Caloric Ratio Measure - Per Serving:

- Kcals: 271.9
- Net Carbohydrates: 1.4 g
- Protein: 48.5 g
- Fat Content: 8.2 g

Ingredients:

- Tilapia fillets (2 @ 5-6 oz./140-170 g each)
- Non-fat plain yogurt (2 tsp.)
- Light mayonnaise (2 tsp.)
- Parmesan cheese (.25 cup - shredded)
- Fresh dill (2-4 sprigs)
- Garlic or powder salt - divided (1 tsp.)
- Black pepper (as desired)
- Non-stick cooking spray (as needed)

Preparation Technique:

1. Set the oven to broil on high.
2. If the fish is frozen, thaw it before cooking.
3. Combine the mayo with parmesan and yogurt in a mixing container till it's incorporated thoroughly.
4. Prepare a baking tray using a layer of aluminum foil and spray it with the cooking spray.
5. Arrange the fillets on the tray - about two inches apart.
6. Portion the cheese mixture - spreading it evenly over the fillets.
7. Dust them using crumbled dill, pepper, and garlic powder/salt to your liking.
8. Arrange the cookie sheet about six inches below the broiler (first rack).

9. Bake for five to seven minutes. Once the cheese starts to brown, check them every ½ minute or so. They're ready when the fish is easily flaked.
   10. Turn the broiler off - leave the tray of fish in the oven (5 min.).
   11. Remove the tray and serve the delicious fish with your preferred side dishes.

Parmesan Shrimp

Servings Provided: 2

Prep & Cook Time: 20 minutes

Caloric Ratio Measure - Per Serving:
- Kcals: 137.6
- Net Carbohydrates: 4.5 g
- Protein: 10.2 g
- Fat Content: 8.6 g

Ingredients:
- Shrimp (14 medium/26-30 per lb. count)
- Olive oil (1 tbsp.)
- Garlic (half of 1 clove)
- Light salt (2 dashes)
- Creole seasoning (.25 tsp.)
- Fresh ground pepper (2 dashes)
- Panko breadcrumbs (.125 cup or 1/8 cup)
- Shredded parmesan cheese (1 tbsp.)
- Optional: Lemon wedges
- Butter-flavored/keto-friendly cooking spray (as needed)
- Also Needed: 8x8 inch/20x20-cm baking pan

Preparation Technique:

1. You can use either - fresh and thawed pre-peeled shrimp. Mince the garlic.
2. Peel and devein the shrimp and toss them into a zipper-type bag with the garlic, olive oil, salt, pepper, and creole seasoning. Gently flip the bag in all directions until the shrimp is well coated.
3. Place the bag in the fridge for 30 minutes to one hour.
4. Warm the oven at 475° Fahrenheit/246° Celsius.
5. Toss the breadcrumbs and parmesan into the baggie and gently turn to coat.
6. Arrange the shrimp into an ungreased pan (single-layered), so they're not touching. Spritz the baking tray using the cooking spray.

7. Broil for approximately ten minutes until done. Serve promptly.
8. Garnish with lemon wedges as desired (add the carbs).
9. Note: The prep time doesn't include ½ hour to marinate or to peel the shrimp.

Salmon Cakes

Servings Provided: 4

Prep & Cook Time: 30 minutes

Caloric Ratio Measure - Per Serving:

- Kcals: 195
- Net Carbohydrates: 3.6 g
- Fat Content: 10 g
- Protein: 23 g

Ingredients:

- Wild Alaskan Pink Salmon/your favorite brand (14.75 oz./420 g can)
- Raw onion (1 cup + more if desired)
- Garlic powder (1 tsp.)
- Large egg (1)
- Black pepper (1 tsp.)
- Salt (as desired)
- Butter or other fat - to fry

Preparation Technique:

1. Mix all of the fixings to form four patties.
2. Fry patties as you would a hamburger in a bit of butter for flavoring.
3. Serve with your favorite sides or in a sandwich.

Shrimp Scampi for Garlic Lovers

Servings Provided: 6

Prep & Cook Time: 15 minutes

Caloric Ratio Measure - Per Serving:

- Kcals: 120.5
- Net Carbohydrates: 1.2 g
- Fat Content: 5.4 g
- Protein: 16 g

Ingredients:

- Frozen - defrosted/fresh shrimp (450 g/1 lb.)
- Garlic (5 cloves + more if desired)
- Olive oil (.125 or 1/8 cup)
- Parsley (2 tbsp. + more for garnish)
- To Serve: Lemon juice (1 lemon + lemon wedges for serving
- Black pepper & salt (1 tsp. each)

Preparation Technique:

1. Warm the oil using the low-temperature setting. Mince and add the garlic and sauté it until golden. Adjust the temperature setting to med-high.
2. Toss in the shrimp, salt, pepper, and parsley - flipping them over once the bottom side is pink.
3. Cook on the second side until pink on the outside and opaque throughout (10 min.).
4. Mix in lemon juice - cook for 30 seconds.
5. Serve promptly with a portion of parsley and lemon wedges.

Tuna Salad & Chives

Servings Provided: 4

Prep & Cook Time: 6-8 minutes

Caloric Ratio Measure - Per Serving:
- Kcals: 235
- Net Carbohydrates: 1 g
- Fat Content: 18 g
- Protein: 20 g

Ingredients:
- Tuna - packed in olive oil (15 oz. or 430 g)
- Mayonnaise (6 tbsp.)
- Chives (2 tbsp.)
- Pepper (.25 tsp.)

Preparation Technique:

1. Drain the tuna and finely chop the chives.
2. Add all of the fixings except the lettuce into a mixing bowl.
3. Toss well. Enjoy as-is or spoon into romaine lettuce leaves.

Poultry

Balsamic Grilled Chicken Breast

Servings Provided: 8
Prep & Cook Time: 50 minutes
Caloric Ratio Measure - Per Serving:

- Kcals: 210
- Net Carbohydrates: 2.6 g
- Protein: 26 g
- Fat Content: 9.8 g

Ingredients:

- Chicken breast - fresh or frozen (8 @ 4 oz. or 110 g each)
- Olive oil (.5 cup)
- Water (1 cup)
- Balsamic vinegar (2 tbsp.)
- Dried onion flakes (4 tsp.)
- Italian seasoning/see recipe ch.1 (3 tsp.)
- Ground mustard (3 tsp.)
- Thyme (2 tsp.)
- Black pepper & salt (2 tsp. each)

Preparation Technique:

1. Whisk the olive oil with balsamic vinegar, thyme, Italian seasoning, pepper, salt, and onion flakes. Pour it into a one-gallon resealable plastic zipper-type bag.
2. Trim the chicken from all fat and bones. Toss it into the bag.
3. Marinate the chicken for at least 30 minutes.
4. Warm the grill. Add the chicken and sear on both sides. Grill it until the meat is white throughout or has an internal temp of 180° Fahrenheit/82° Celsius.

Blackened Chicken Alfredo Bake

Servings Provided: 8

Prep & Cook Time: 50 minutes

Caloric Ratio Measure - Per Serving:
- Kcals: 240.1
- Net Carbohydrates: 5.7 g
- Fat Content: 12 g
- Protein: 26.9 g

Ingredients:
- Chicken breasts (3)
- Cooking oil (1 tbsp.)
- Yellow squash (1 cup)
- Sweet onion (1 medium)
- Cauliflower (1 cup)
- Montreal Steak Seasoning (to taste)
- Black pepper & salt
- Alfredo sauce (1 jar - 1 lb./ 0.09 oz. size/as desired)
- Grated parmesan cheese (.25 cup)
- Breadcrumbs (.125 or 1/8 cup)
- Also Needed: 13x9/33-23-cm pan

Preparation Technique:

1. Warm the oven at 350° Fahrenheit/177° Celsius.
2. Lightly mist the pan using a spritz of cooking oil spray.
3. Trim the fat and bone from the chicken.
4. Sprinkle the chicken using the steak seasoning - cook in a skillet till it's cooked as desired.
5. Chop and toss the cauliflower in a microwavable dish and add two tablespoons of water. Cover the container using a plastic wrap layer - cook using the high-temperature setting (4 min.).
6. Add oil to the same skillet. Dice and add the onions to sauté until clear.
7. Cube and add the squash with pepper and salt to sauté until softened.
8. Dice the cooled chicken into cubes and add to the baking dish

with the veggies and sauce. Top it off using breadcrumbs and cheese.

9. Set a timer to bake for 20 minutes. Switch to the broil setting until the top is nicely browned (10 min.).

Chicken & Cheese Stuffed Peppers

Servings Provided: 8 @ ½ pepper
each **Prep & Cook Time**: 45 minutes
Caloric Ratio Measure - Per Serving:

- Kcals: 325
- Net Carbohydrates: 5 g
- Fat Content: 25 g
- Protein: 20 g

Ingredients:

- Green poblano/bell peppers (4 large/656 g)
- Shredded chicken breast (3 cups/420 g)
- Mayonnaise (.5 cup)
- Cream cheese (4 tbsp.)
- Olive oil (5 tbsp.)
- Shredded cheddar cheese (.5 cup)
- Salsa Verde (8 oz./230 g)

- Fresh or pickled jalapenos
- Crumbled pork rinds
- Cilantro
- Cajun Seasoning

Preparation Technique:

1. Heat the oven temperature at 425° Fahrenheit/218° Celsius.
2. Slice the peppers into halves - lengthwise and trash the seeds. Arrange the halves with the cut side facing upward in a baking dish.
3. Shred and combine the chicken with the mayo, cream cheese, and optional fixings as desired. Add extra salsa verde if desired, but add the carbs. Sprinkle using a sprinkle of pepper and salt.
4. Stuff the peppers using the chicken mixture.
5. Generously spritz the peppers using the oil and top them off using the shredded cheese. Crumble the pork rinds over the top if desired.
6. Bake the peppers until they are done as desired (20 min. to ½

hr.).

1.

Chicken Nuggets

Servings Provided: 24 nuggets @ 6
servings **Prep & Cook Time**: 45 minutes
Caloric Ratio Measure - Per Serving:
- Kcals: 2124
- Net Carbohydrates: 11 g
- Protein: 65 g
- Fat Content: 203 g

Ingredients:
- Chicken breast (2 cups)
- Coconut flour (.25 cup)
- Avocado oil (.5 cup)
- Mayonnaise (.5 cup)
- Fresh egg (1 large/50 g)
- Salt/pepper (as desired)

Preparation Technique:

1. Finely shred and combine the chicken with the coconut flour and seasonings. Use a fork to combine the fixings, evenly distributing and coating the chicken with the dry components.
2. Fold in avocado oil, mayo, and egg. Stir to combine until it's similar to a pancake mix.
3. Warm a skillet using the med-high temperature setting (about 450° Fahrenheit to 232° Celsius).
4. Drop spoonfuls of the batter and fry as you would pancakes, flipping at least once.
5. Once the nuggets have thoroughly cooked, leave them in the pan to cool and absorb the oil, or scrape the pan and drizzle the oil over the nuggets.
6. Serve them promptly or freeze them in a single layer - adding them to a freezer container or plastic bag.
7. To reheat, place the frozen nuggets in a pan and heat until thawed using the med-low temperature setting.

8. Alternatively, warm the oven to reach 450° Fahrenheit/232° Celsius.
9. Bake the nuggets in cupcake tins for about 15 to 20 minutes. Cool in the molds to reabsorb fat that has cooked out.

Creamy Chicken Broccoli

Servings Provided: 1

Prep & Cook Time: 26 minutes

Caloric Ratio Measure - Per Serving:

- Kcals: 50
- Net Carbohydrates: 5 g
- Fat Content: 46 g
- Protein: 18 g

Ingredients:

- 36% heavy cream/see recipe ch.1 (40 g or 1/3 cup)
- Broccoli - raw (80 g/approx. 1 cup)
- Lemon juice 100% - bottled or fresh (1 tsp.)
- Large chicken breast (70 g - about 1/3 of a breast)
- Butter (2 tbsp.)
- Olive oil (1.5 tbsp.)
- For Thinning: Chicken broth - 100% Natural
- Optional: Tabasco sauce (to your liking)

Preparation Technique:

1. Heat a skillet using a med-high temperature setting to melt the butter with olive oil.
2. Carefully trim the chicken into bite-sized chunks and add it to the pan. Sauté for three minutes, turning the chicken to brown.
3. Reduce the temperature to medium. Mix in the lemon juice, a dash of black pepper, Tabasco sauce, and salt - stirring until coated.
4. Chop the broccoli into bite-sized pieces. Stir in cream and broccoli. Simmer for two to three more minutes while stirring.
5. Mix in the chicken broth and cover the pan. Turn off the burner - let it rest about ten minutes to finish cooking the broccoli and chicken.

Feta Chicken Burgers

Servings Provided: 4 patties **Prep & Cook Time**: 20 minutes **Caloric Ratio Measure - Per Serving**:

- Kcals: 285.6
- Net Carbohydrates: 2.5 g
- Protein: 26.8 g
- Fat Content: 19.8 g

Ingredients:

- Ground chicken (450 g/1 lb.)
- Crumbled feta (170 g/6 oz.)
- Ground oregano (1 tbsp.)
- Garlic powder & salt (.25 tsp. each)

Preparation Technique:

1. Warm either an outside grill or the oven broiler.
2. Mix each of the fixings to make four individual patties.
3. Cook the meat till done or have an internal temp of 165° Fahrenheit/74° Celsius (7-8 min. per side).

Fiesta Lime Chicken

Servings Provided: 8 @ ½ breast each

Prep & Cook Time: 17-20 minutes

Caloric Ratio Measure - Per Serving:

- Kcals: 209
- Net Carbohydrates: 5.6 g
- Fat Content: 6.2 g
- Protein: 31.4 g

Ingredients:

- Chicken breast (4)
- Garlic (3 cloves)
- Juice (1½ limes)
- Salsa (1 cup)
- Reduced-fat ranch dressing (.25 cup)
- Cheddar cheese - reduced-fat (1 cup - shredded)

Preparation Technique:

1. Trim the chicken, making sure all fat and bones are removed to slice them into halves.
2. Lightly spritz a skillet with cooking oil spray and heat using the medium-temperature setting.
3. Sauté the chicken for three minutes on each side. Mince and toss in the garlic.
4. Whisk the salsa, lime juice, and ranch dressing in a mixing container. Spread it over the top of the chicken. Simmer for an additional five minutes.
5. Garnish it with the cheese, cover, and cook till the chicken is done (4-5 min.).

Parmesan Chicken

Servings Provided: 1
Prep & Cook Time: 35 minutes
Caloric Ratio Measure - Per Serving:
- Kcals: 190.6
- Net Carbohydrates: 0.4 g
- Fat Content: 7 g
- Protein: 29.2 g

Ingredients:
- Chicken breast (1)
- Dijon mustard (1 tsp.)
- Grated parmesan cheese (2 tbsp.)
- Cooking oil spray (as needed)

Preparation Technique:

1. Trim the fat and bones from the chicken breasts.
2. Brush the chicken with the dijon mustard evenly on both sides.
3. Pat cheese onto the chicken to create a crust.
4. Arrange it on a baking tray. Lightly spritz it using the cooking spray to help make it golden brown and crusty.
5. Bake at 375° Fahrenheit/191° Celsius for 20 to 30 minutes and serve as desired.

Quick & Easy Creamy Mushroom Chicken

Servings Provided: 6

Prep & Cook Time: 45 minutes

Caloric Ratio Measure - Per Serving:
- Kcals: 224
- Net Carbohydrates: 5.8 g
- Fat Content: 7.9 g
- Protein: 29.7 g

Ingredients:
- Boneless & skinless chicken breast or tenderloins - diced (1.5 lb./680 g)
- Low-sodium chicken broth (2 cups)
- Cream of chicken/mushroom soup (2 small cans)
- Neufchatel low-fat cream cheese (3 oz./85 g)
- Fresh chives (4 tbsp.) or (can use dry also)
- Mushrooms - drained (1 cup - canned)

Preparation Technique:

1. Drain the mushrooms and set them aside.
2. Prepare a large - high-sided skillet with the broth and diced chicken breast.
3. Set the temperature to high. Once boiling, adjust the temperature setting to med-high and continue cooking chicken, occasionally stirring, for about ½ hour until it's no longer pink inside and tender.
4. Mix in the cream of mushroom soup, mushrooms, and Neufchatel cream cheese. Mix well until cream cheese is melted and all of the fixings are incorporated, and the mixture is hot (5-10 min.)
5. Serve as is or with a serving of noodles or rice.

Ranch-Baked Chicken

Servings Provided: 6
Prep & Cook Time: 60 minutes
Caloric Ratio Measure - Per Serving:
- Kcals: 191.2
- Net Carbohydrates: 1.2 g
- Fat Content: 16.1 g
- Protein: 9.5 g

Ingredients:
- Chicken breast (6 - bone-in)
- Creamy Ranch dressing (1 cup)
- Seasoning salt (2 tsp.)
- Crushed basil leaves - dry (1 tsp.)
- Pepper (1 tsp.)
- Also Needed: 9x13/23x33-cm baking dish

Preparation Technique:

1. Set the oven temperature at 425° Fahrenheit/218° Celsius.
2. Rinse chicken breast and arrange it in the baking dish,
3. Season each of the chicken breasts with basil, pepper, and seasoning salt.
4. Add the dressing to the chicken and cover the baking dish with a layer of foil.
5. Set a timer to bake it for 45 minutes and serve.

Rosemary & Olive Oil Slow Cooked Chicken

Servings Provided: 8 @ 4 oz. each.
Prep & Cook Time: 2 hours 50 minutes
Caloric Ratio Measure - Per Serving:

- Kcals: 192.1
- Net Carbohydrates: 1.1 g
- Protein: 26 g
- Fat Content: 8.2 g

Ingredients:

- Garlic - sliced (8 cloves)
- Dried rosemary crumbled between your fingers (1 tbsp.)
- Back pepper & kosher salt (.5 tsp.)
- E-V olive oil (3 tbsp.)
- Water (2 tbsp.)
- White wine (3 tbsp.)
- Chicken breasts (910 g/2 lb.)
- Baking spray (as needed)

Preparation Technique:

1. Spray a slow cooker with a spritz of cooking spray.
2. Trim the fat and bones from the chicken.
3. Toss all the fixings (not the chicken) into the cooker.
4. Place each chicken piece in the cooker making sure they are thoroughly covered with the mixture.
5. Set a timer using the low setting (8 hrs.) or set it to high for a quicker cooking time (4 hrs.).
6. Serve it with couscous or rice and your favorite steamed veggies.
7. Leftovers (if you have any) are an excellent option for a salad or pasta dish the next day.

Spinach - Cheese & Ham-Stuffed Chicken Breast

Servings Provided: 4
Prep & Cook Time: 40 minutes
Caloric Ratio Measure - Per Serving:

- Kcals: 271.4
- Net Carbohydrates: 5.6 g
- Protein: 39.6 g
- Fat Content: 8.7 g

Ingredients:

- Chicken breasts (4 @ 4 oz./110 g each)
- Low-sodium ham (4 slices @ 1 oz./28 g each)
- Fat-free mozzarella cheese (4 slices @ 1 oz./28 g each)
- Baby spinach leaves (1 cup)
- A-P flour - divided (4 tbsp.)
- E-V olive oil (1 tbsp.)
- Keto-friendly butter spread (1 tbsp.)
- Chicken broth - 99% fat-free (1 cup)
- Heavy cream/see recipe ch.1 (1 tbsp.)
- Black pepper and salt (as desired)

Preparation Technique:

1. Heat the oven at 350° Fahrenheit/177° Celsius.
2. Rinse and chop the spinach leaves, and set aside.
3. Remove the fat and skin from the chicken. Slice each breast horizontally, almost to the opposite edge - fold back the top half. Lightly dust using pepper and salt.
4. Place one slice each of ham and mozzarella and ¼ cup spinach on each check breast. Fold the top half of the breasts over the filling.
5. Scatter flour (3 tbsp.) on a plate. Hold the breasts closed and cover them with the flour and a dusting of pepper and salt. Shake off the excess.
6. Warm the oil and butter spread in a big frying pan using a medium-temperature setting. Arrange the chicken in the skillet - fry it till it's nicely browned (4 min. per side).

7. Scoop the fried chicken to a shallow baking dish.
8. Bake till chicken the juices run clear when poked with a fork - the center should not be pink (10 min.).
9. Whisk the cream with the chicken broth and the rest of the flour (1 tbsp.) in a mixing container.
10. Pour the broth mixture into the chicken's skillet and warm it using the medium-temperature setting, constantly stirring, until the sauce thickens (3 min.).
11. Serve the chicken with the fresh sauce over the top to serve.

Lamb Favorites

Lamb & Asparagus With Tangy Sauce

Servings Provided: 1
Prep & Cook Time: 30 minutes
Caloric Ratio Measure - Per Serving:

- Kcals: 500
- Net Carbohydrates: 3.7 g
- Protein: 15 g
- Fat Content: 47 g

Ingredients:

- Olive oil (1 tbsp.)
- Orange juice - unsweetened (1 tsp.)
- Lime juice - unsweetened (1 tsp.)
- Garlic (1 minced clove)
- Curry powder (1 tsp.)
- Raw lamb shoulder (2.8 oz./80 g)
- Asparagus - raw (.5 cup)

Preparation Technique:

1. Mince and add the garlic with the curry powder, orange juice, and lime juice to make the marinade.
2. Cut a one-inch slice of lamb shoulder to the appropriate servings size for one serving and place it in a small bowl with the marinade sauce. Pop it into the fridge for two to four hours.
3. Use an eight-inch square piece of foil and place it on a shallow oven-proof dish. Arrange the lamb on the foil and surround it with the asparagus spears. Broil it for six to eight minutes - rotating it once. Remove the asparagus as they are browned.
4. Meanwhile, prepare a saucepan to warm the oil.
5. Add in the marinade to simmer till it's thickened. Transfer the cooked asparagus and lamb to the pan and turn off the heat. Wait a few minutes and serve.

Roasted Leg of Lamb

Servings Provided: 6

Prep & Cook Time: 2 hours - varies

Caloric Ratio Measure - Per Serving:
- Net Carbohydrates: 1 g
- Kcals: 223
- Fat Content: 14 g
- Protein: 22 g

Ingredients:
- Reduced-sodium beef broth (.5 cup)
- Leg of lamb (2 lb./910 g)
- Chopped garlic cloves (6)
- Fresh rosemary leaves (1 tbsp.)
- Black pepper (1 tsp.)

Preparation Technique:

1. Grease a baking pan and set the oven temperature to 400° Fahrenheit/204° Celsius.
2. Arrange the lamb in the pan and add the broth and seasonings.
3. Roast for 30 minutes and lower the heat to 350° Fahrenheit/177° Celsius. Continue cooking for about one hour or until done.
4. Let the lamb stand about 20 minutes before slicing to serve.
5. Enjoy with some roasted brussels sprouts and extra rosemary for a tasty change of pace.

Other Dinnertime Favorites

Asian Cabbage Stir-Fry

Servings Provided: 4
Prep & Cook Time: 55 minutes
Caloric Ratio Measure - Per Serving:

- Kcals: 841
- Net Carbohydrates: 9 g
- Fat Content: 74 g
- Protein: 30 g

Ingredients:

- Green cabbage (1 lb./450 g)
- Butter or coconut oil - divided (2 oz./56 g)
- Salt (1 tsp.)
- Black pepper (.25 tsp.)
- Onion powder (1 tsp.)
- White wine vinegar (1 tbsp.)
- Chili flakes (1 tsp.)
- Garlic (2 cloves)
- Fresh ginger (2 oz./9.66 tbsp./56 g)
- Ground beef or ground turkey (1.25 lb./570 g)
- Scallions (3 @ 1.5 oz./42 g)
- Sesame oil (1 tbsp.)

- Mayonnaise (1 cup)
- Wasabi paste (.5 tbsp.)

Preparation Technique:

1. Finely shred the cabbage and fry it using half of the butter in a big skillet/wok using a med-high temperature setting till it is softened.
2. Add spices and vinegar - stir and fry for a couple of minutes more and scoop the cabbage into a holding container.
3. Melt the rest of the butter in the same skillet. Mince and add ginger, garlic, and chili flakes to sauté for a few minutes.

4. Mix in the meat and brown until most of the juices have evaporated. Lower the temperature setting - slightly.
5. Chop and add scallions (cut into 1.5-cm/0.5 inches) and cabbage to the meat.
6. Stir until it's piping hot with a dusting of salt and pepper. Drizzle with sesame oil before serving.
7. Mix the wasabi mayonnaise - starting with a small amount of wasabi and adding more until the flavor is to your liking.
8. Serve the stir-fry warm with a scoop of wasabi mayonnaise over its top.

Asian-Inspired Pork Chops

Servings Provided: 3

Prep & Cook Time: 20 minutes

Caloric Ratio Measure - Per Serving:

- Kcals: 106
- Net Carbohydrates: 2.7 g
- Fat Content: 5.5 g
- Protein: 11.5 g

Ingredients:

- Pork chops (3 thinly sliced - center-cut)
- Salt (1 dash)
- Liquid Aminos/Sub. for soy sauce/or another favorite keto-friendly (2 tbsp.)
- Garlic powder (.5 tsp.)
- Ginger (.5 tsp.)
- Black pepper (.5 tsp.)
- Garlic (2 tsp.)
- Onions (1 tbsp.)

Preparation Technique:

1. Mince the garlic and dice the onions. Toss everything into a zipper-type plastic bag. Shake the fixings.
2. Put the pork chops in a bag. Marinate for two to 24 hours in the fridge, turning the bag from time to time.
3. Discard the marinade and drain the meat.
4. Grill them for 12-15 minutes using the medium temperature setting or until the desired doneness.

Beef Stroganoff

Servings Provided: 1

Prep & Cook Time: minutes

Caloric Ratio Measure - Per Serving:
- Kcals: 447
- Net Carbohydrates: 6 g
- Fat Content: 28 g
- Protein: 39 g

Ingredients:
- Lean ground beef (1 lb. or 450 g)
- Sliced mushrooms (8 oz. or 230 g)
- Minced cloves of garlic (2)
- Butter (2 tbsp.)
- Sour cream (1.25 cups)
- Lemon juice (1 tsp.)
- Water or dry white wine (.33 cup)
- Dried parsley (1 tsp.)
- Paprika (.25 tsp.)
- *Optional:* Freshly chopped parsley (1 tbsp.)

Preparation Technique:

1. Warm a skillet to sauté the onions and garlic using one tablespoon of butter.
2. Mix the beef into the pan, and sprinkle with pepper and salt if desired. Cook until done and set to the side.
3. Add the remainder of the butter, mushrooms, and the wine/water to the pan.
4. Cook until half of the liquid is reduced and the mushrooms are soft.
5. Take them away from the heat and add the paprika and sour cream.
6. On low heat, stir in the meat and lemon juice. Use additional spices for flavoring if desired.

Crockpot Pork Chops

Servings Provided: 10

Prep & Cook Time: 7-9 hours/varies

Caloric Ratio Measure - Per Serving:

- Kcals: 239.7
- Net Carbohydrates: 7.7 g
- Fat Content: 12.1 g
- Protein: 21.8 g

Ingredients:

- Pork chops (Family pack - about 10)
- Low-sodium/low-fat cream/mushroom/chicken.celery, etc. (1 can)
- Ketchup (.5 cup)

Preparation Technique:

1. Arrange the chops in the cooker. Add the ketchup and soup of choice.
2. Stir and close the lid. Place the timer on for seven to nine hours on the low setting.

Hot Tex-Mex Pork Casserole

Servings Provided: 4

Prep & Cook Time: 35 minutes

Caloric Ratio Measure - Per Serving:

- Kcals: 431
- Net Carbohydrates: 7.8 g
- Protein: 43 g
- Fat Content: 24 g

Ingredients:

- Butter (2 tbsp.)
- Pork - ground (1.5 lb./680 g)
- Tex-Mex/another spicy seasoning (3 tbsp.)
- Jalapenos (2 tbsp.)
- Monterey jack shredded cheese (.5 cup)
- Crushed tomatoes (.5 cup)

- Scallion (1)
- Sour cream (1 cup)

Preparation Technique:

1. Warm the oven to reach 330° Fahrenheit/166° Celsius.
2. Lightly spritz a baking tray using a cooking oil spray.
3. Prepare a skillet - add the butter and pork to cook till browned (8 min.). Add the jalapenos, Tex-Mex, pepper, salt, and tomatoes. Simmer it for about five minutes.
4. Dump the fixings into the prepared dish and drizzle it with the cheese.
5. Set the timer for 20 minutes until it's golden brown.
6. Garnish as desired.

Keto Pizza Chaffles

Servings Provided: 4

Prep & Cook Time: 15 minutes

Caloric Ratio Measure - Per Serving:

- Kcals: 421
- Net Carbohydrates: 3 g
- Fat Content: 33 g
- Protein: 27 g

Ingredients:

The Chaffles:

- Eggs (4)
- Shredded cheddar cheese (8 oz./2 cups/230 g)
- Italian seasoning (.5 tsp.)
- Parmesan cheese - grated (1 oz./28 g)

- Tomato sauce - sugar-free (4 tsp.)
- Pepperoni (16 slices)
- Shredded mozzarella cheese (.75 cup/3 oz./85 g)

Preparation Technique:

1. Warm your waffle maker.
2. Combine each of the fixings in a mixing bowl and thoroughly whisk.
3. Lightly grease the waffle maker - evenly spoon the mixture over the bottom plate, spreading it out slightly. Close the waffle iron and cook (approx 6 min. depending on your model).
4. Gently lift the lid when you believe they're done.
5. Cover a large baking tray using a layer of parchment baking paper and place the chaffles on it.
6. Spread each chaffle with tomato sauce and top with pepperoni slices and mozzarella.
7. Place under a hot grill until the cheese is browned and bubbly (approx. 2 min.).
8. Note: The chaffles are best eaten straight away but can be frozen and reheated. They can also be stored, wrapped well, in the

fridge for up to four days for lunch prep.

Maple Country-Style Pork Ribs - Slow-Cooked

Servings Provided: 4

Prep & Cook Time: 7-9 hours

Caloric Ratio Measure - Per Serving:
- Kcals: 188.4
- Net Carbohydrates: 2 g
- Protein: 22.3 g
- Fat Content: 9.4 g

Ingredients:
- Ground allspice (.25 tsp.)
- Ground cinnamon (.25 tsp.)
- Country-style pork ribs (2 lb./910 g before cooking - will yield 16 oz./450 g meat)
- Onion (.25 cup)
- Garlic powder (.5 tsp.)
- Maple-flavored syrup- no sugar (1 tbsp.)
- Black pepper (1 dash)
- Ground ginger (.25 tsp.)
- Low-sodium soy sauce (1 tbsp.)

Preparation Technique:

1. Dice the onion and measure the rest of the components. Toss all of the fixings except for the ribs into a mixing container.
2. Pour the sauce over the ribs.
3. Pop it into a crockpot, close the lid, and set the timer for seven to nine hours (on low).

Sausage Sheet Pan Dinner

Servings Provided: 4

Prep & Cook Time: 30 minutes

Caloric Ratio Measure - Per Serving:

- Kcals: 506
- Net Carbohydrates: 7 g
- Fat Content: 43 g
- Protein: 19 g

Ingredients:

- Smoked sausage (1 lb. or 450 g)
- Yellow bell pepper (1)
- Broccoli florets (4 cups)
- Radishes (1 cup)
- Onion (.5 cup)
- Olive oil (2 tbsp.)
- Salt (1 tsp.)
- Black pepper (.5 tsp.)
- Italian seasoning/see recipe ch.1 (1 tsp.)
- Fresh basil (1 tbsp.)

Preparation Technique:

1. Set the oven temperature to 400° Fahrenheit/204° Celsius.
2. Cover a rimmed sheet pan with foil.
3. Slice the radishes into halves.
4. Slice and toss the sausage, bell pepper, broccoli, radishes, and onions into the pan.
5. Drizzle the olive oil over the pan, then sprinkle with the salt, Italian seasoning, and black pepper. Toss everything thoroughly.
6. Bake the pan for 20 minutes.
7. Divide the sausage and veggies between plates - sprinkle with the freshly chopped basil.
8. Enjoy while it's hot.

Chapter 5: Ketogenic Side Dish Recipes

Bacon-Wrapped Brussel Sprouts

Servings Provided: 12

Prep & Cook Time: 45 minutes

Caloric Ratio Measure - Per Serving:
- Kcals: 58
- Net Carbohydrates: 1 g
- Fat Content: 4 g
- Protein: 4 g

Ingredients:
- Bacon (12 strips)
- Brussel sprouts (12 medium-large)
- Black pepper (to your liking)

Preparation Technique:

1. Set the oven temperature at 375° Fahrenheit/191° Celsius.
2. Prepare a baking tray using a layer of foil.
3. Rinse and dry the sprouts using a paper towel.
4. Place the sprout on a slice of bacon and roll it until covered. Arrange them on the baking tray and season to your liking.
5. Bake them for 30 to 35 minutes. Serve using a toothpick as a handle.

Cabbage Patties

Servings Provided: 8 patties - 4
servings **Prep & Cook Time**: 25 minutes
Caloric Ratio Measure - Per Serving:

- Net Carbohydrates: 1 g
- Fat Content: 4 g
- Protein: 1 g

Ingredients:

- Cabbage (3 cups) or Egg (1 large)
- Coconut flour (.75 tbsp.)
- Coconut oil - melted (2 tbsp.)
- Optional: Garlic powder & salt

Preparation Technique:

1. Cook and finely chop the cabbage. Toss it with the seasonings and flour into a food processor. Pulse three to four times or until the coconut flour is evenly dispersed.
2. Crack the egg into the mixture and add the oil. Pulse it for another three to four pulses to combine thoroughly. Don't the cabbage too fine.
3. Roll the mixture into eight balls and flatten.
4. Lightly spray a skillet with a cooking oil spray or add additional fat. Add the patties and cook until done.
5. Serve the patties plain or top it off as desired - but count the carbs.

Cool & Spicy Jicama Slaw

Servings Provided: 8

Prep & Cook Time: 8-10 minutes

Caloric Ratio Measure - Per Serving:
- Net Carbohydrates: 3 g
- Fat Content: 7 g
- Protein: 1 g

Ingredients:
- Julienned jicama (200 g/4 cups)
- Avocado (200 g/1 large)
- Julienned cucumber (200 g/4 cups)
- Radish - sliced thinly (50 g/2 large)
- Grapeseed oil (25 g/2 tbsp.)
- Lime juice (from 1 large lime/25 g/2 tbsp.)
- Optional: Red chili pepper flakes (as desired)

Preparation Technique:

1. Use the widest julienne setting to prepare the jicama and cucumber. Weigh or measure and combine each in a large mixing container.
2. Use the thinnest setting to slice the radish and toss them with the cucumbers.
3. Prepare the juice by squeezing the lime and straining any seeds from the juice. Dice the avocado and toss in the juice until coated to help prevent the avocado from premature browning.
4. Toss the avocado with the veggies.
5. If you prefer a creamier slaw, mash the avocado with the juice until smooth, and add the avocado mixture to the jicama. Pour the oil over the mixture, tossing to combine.
6. If using, mix in the chili flakes and wait about ½ hour before serving.

Garlic & Olive Oil Spaghetti Squash

Servings Provided: 2 - main meal or 4 - sides **Prep & Cook Time**: 6 minutes

Caloric Ratio Measure - Per Serving:
- Kcals: 181.4
- Net Carbohydrates: 11.6 g
- Protein: 1.7 g
- Fat Content: 14.5 g

Ingredients:
- Spaghetti squash (1)
- Garlic (3-4 cloves)
- Olive oil (2 tbsp.)
- Water (.25 cup)
- Salt and pepper (to your liking)

Preparation Technique:

1. Warm the oven to reach 375° Fahrenheit/191° Celsius.
2. Slice the squash in half - lengthwise. Scoop out seeds, saving as much of the inside as possible.
3. Prepare a casserole with a bit of cooking oil spray. Place the squash face-down, and add the water.
4. Bake for ½ hour. Flip the squash and continue cooking for an additional ½ hour - until softened.
5. Add oil to a pan. Mince and sauté the garlic. Grab a serving fork to scrape the squash into the pan to finish cooking (3-5 min.).
6. Serve it with a shake of pepper and salt.

Lavender & Butter Braised Celery

Servings Provided: 2

Prep & Cook Time: 30 minutes

Caloric Ratio Measure - Per Serving:

- Net Carbohydrates: 2 g
- Fat Content: 12 g
- Protein: 1 g

Ingredients:

- Celery heart (1 @ 10.6 oz./300 g)
- Butter (28 g/2 tbsp.)
- Herbs-de-Provence with lavender (1 pinch)
- Water

Preparation Technique:

1. Trim the celery and rinse under cold water.
2. Use a vegetable peeler to peel the largest stalks of celery.
3. Measure and add the butter, herbs, and celery into an oversized skillet. Fill the pan with water to cover halfway up the celery's sides.
4. Wait for the water to boil down (75% reduction), and simmer the celery until it's tender and the sauce is creamy.
5. Portion as desired to serve.
6. *Note*: Taste test before adding salt if you used regular butter.

Mock Potato Casserole

Servings Provided: 8

Prep & Cook Time: 50 minutes

Caloric Ratio Measure - Per Serving:

- Kcals: 164.6
- Net Carbohydrates: 1.6 g
- Fat Content: 11.7 g
- Protein: 10.8 g

Ingredients:

- Frozen cauliflower (16 oz./450 g bag)
- Light butter with canola oil - spreadable (2 tbsp.)
- Unchilled cream cheese (4 oz./110 g)
- Turkey bacon - cooked until crispy & crumbled (1 lb./450 g)
- Shredded sharp cheddar cheese - divided (8 oz./230 g)
- Chopped green onions or parsley (2 tbsp.)
- Water (2 tbsp.)

Preparation Technique:

1. Warm the oven temperature to reach 350° Fahrenheit/177° Celsius.
2. Lightly spritz a casserole dish.
3. Microwave cauliflower with the water for 10 to 15 minutes until softened, drain, and mash using a potato masher.
4. Blend in the cream cheese and butter.
5. Add the shredded cheese (setting aside about ½ cup) and the rest of the fixings.
6. Scoop it into the prepared dish - topping it off using the last portion of cheese.
7. Bake until brown and bubbly (20 min.).

Roasted Salt & Pepper Radish Chips

Servings Provided: 4

Prep & Cook Time: 25 minutes

Caloric Ratio Measure - Per Serving:
- Kcals: 70
- Net Carbohydrates: 1.2 g
- Fat Content: 7.1 g
- Protein: 0.4 g

Ingredients:
- Fresh radishes (16 oz./450 g)
- Melted coconut/olive oil (2 tbsp.)
- Black pepper and sea salt (.5 tsp. of each)

Preparation Technique:

1. Warm the oven to reach 400° Fahrenheit/204° Celsius.
2. Use a mandolin to thinly slice the radishes. Place them in a container and toss them with the oil.
3. Layer them onto two baking trays, not overlapping, and dust with the pepper and salt.
4. Bake for 12 to 15 minutes and serve when ready.

Shortcut Smoky Collard Greens

Servings Provided: 6

Prep & Cook Time: 1.5 hours

Caloric Ratio Measure - Per Serving:

- Kcals: 184
- Net Carbohydrates: 4 g
- Protein: 3.6 g
- Fat Content: 17 g

Ingredients:

- Butter (.25 cup)
- Roasted beef bone marrow (.25 cup)
- Yellow onion (1 cup/115 g)
- Collard greens - stems & leaves (680 g/1.5 lb.)
- Garlic (3 cloves/9 g)
- Smoked paprika (1 tbsp./6.8 g)
- Salt (as desired)

Preparation Technique:

1. Use a stockpot to melt the butter and bone marrow using the med-high temperature setting.
2. Slice and toss the onion into the pot to sauté till it's softened.
3. Mince or chop the garlic and collards, and add them with smoked paprika and salt to the cooking pot.
4. Toss the collards until they begin to wilt. Then, pour in water to fill about one-third of the way up the sides of the greens.
5. Adjust the temperature until it's simmering, not a full boil.
6. Braise the greens in the water until the stems' thickest segments are tender or until most of the water has evaporated (20 min.).
7. Transfer the greens to a mixing container and garnish with more paprika as desired.

Zucchini Noodle Gratin

Servings Provided: 8

Prep & Cook Time: 1 hour 45 minutes

Caloric Ratio Measure - Per Serving:

- Kcals: 200
- Net Carbohydrates: 3 g
- Fat Content: 18 g
- Protein: 6 g

Ingredients:

- Loosely packed zucchini noodles (8 cups/800 g)
- Heavy cream (1 cup/238 g)
- Shredded Gruyere cheese (113 g/4 oz.)
- Butter (42 g/3 tbsp.)

- Black pepper
- Salt
- Garlic powder
- Fresh herbs
- Also Needed: 9-inch/23-cm baking dish

Preparation Technique:

1. Make the zucchini noodles and place them in a mesh colander. Grab and garnish using the salt and toss to coat evenly. Leave them in the sink for about two hours to release moisture. Gently dry and squeeze the surplus moisture from the noodles using several paper towels.
2. Warm the oven to reach 350° Fahrenheit/177° Celsius.
3. Lightly grease the baking dish with butter and add the noodles in an even layer.
4. Use a saucepan to combine the butter, heavy cream, and cheese. Warm the mixture using the medium-temperature setting until melted and the sauce is smooth. Transfer the pan to a cool burner and add optional seasonings.
5. Scoop the cream sauce evenly over the noodles - bake for about one hour or until nicely browned.

6. Cool the gratin for about 15 minutes and slice it into eight portions to serve.

Chapter 6: Ketogenic Dessert & Snack Recipes

You will love these delicious treats!

Desserts

Baked Goat Cheese With Roasted Pistachios & Blackberries

Servings Provided: 4
Prep & Cook Time: 22-25 minutes
Caloric Ratio Measure - Per Serving:
- Kcals: 584
- Net Carbohydrates: 4 g
- Fat Content: 46 g
- Protein: 33 g

Ingredients:
- Goat cheese (1.25 lb./570 g) *The Sauce*:
- Fresh blackberries (9 oz./260)
- Optional: Erythritol (1 tbsp.)
- Ground cinnamon (1 pinch) *The Topping*:
- Pistachio nuts (1 oz./28 g)
- Fresh rosemary
- Salt

Preparation Technique:

1. Set the oven temperature to 350° Fahrenheit/177° Celsius.
2. Combine the blackberries with cinnamon and sweetener - if using and set aside.
3. Bake the goat cheese in the oven until it gets some color (10-12 min.). Remove and let sit for a few minutes.
4. Roughly chop the pistachios and roast them in a dry skillet - dusting with salt.
5. Top the goat cheese with blackberry, roasted pistachio, and rosemary.

Chocolate Roll Cake

Servings Provided: 12

Prep & Cook Time: 30 minutes

Caloric Ratio Measure - Per Serving:

- Kcals: 275
- Net Carbohydrates: 3 grams
- Protein: 5 grams
- Fat Content: 25 grams

Ingredients:

The Mix:

- Almond flour (1 cup)
- Melted butter (4 tbsp.)
- Eggs (3)
- Psyllium husk powder (.25 cup)
- Cocoa powder (.25 cup)
- Baking powder (1 tsp.)
- Coconut milk (.25 cup)
- Sour cream (.25 cup)
- Erythritol (.25 cup)
- Vanilla (1 tsp.)

- Cream cheese (230 g or 8 oz. pkg.)
- Butter (8 tbsp.)
- Sour cream (.25 cup)
- Erythritol (.25 cup)
- Stevia (.25 cup)
- Vanilla (1 tsp.)

Preparation Technique:

1. Set the oven to reach 350° Fahrenheit/177° Celsius.
2. Combine the dry fixings and combine slowly with the wet components.
3. Mix well and spread the dough over a foil-covered baking tin.
4. Bake it for 12 to 15 minutes. Transfer the pan to the counter to cool slightly to handle.

5. Prepare the filling. Spread the mixture over the dough and roll up the cake. Be sure to make it tight and serve.

Coconut-Caramel Bread

Servings Provided: 10

Preparation & Cooking Time: 1 hour 15-20 minutes

Caloric Ratio Measure - Per Serving:

- Kcals: 265
- Net Carbohydrates: 3 g
- Fat Content: 27 g
- Protein: 3 g

Ingredients:

- Butter - softened (.75 cup)
- Eggs (2)
- Riced cauliflower (1 cup)
- Coconut flour (2 tbsp.)
- Bak. soda (1 tsp.)
- Vanilla extract (1 tsp.)
- Granular erythritol (.5 cup)
- Pumpkin puree (.5 cup) *The Topping*:
- Coconut milk (1 can)
- Granular erythritol (.25 cup)
- Toasted & shredded unsweetened coconut (.5 cup)

Preparation Technique:

1. Warm the oven to reach 350° Fahrenheit/177° Celsius and grease a loaf pan.
2. Mix the eggs, butter, and cauliflower in a large mixing container till it is entirely incorporated.
3. Add the coconut flour, baking soda, vanilla extract, erythritol, and pumpkin to the bowl and stir well.
4. Scoop the batter into the prepared pan and bake until a toothpick comes out of the center cleanly (40-50 min.).
5. Meanwhile, make the caramel topping by combining the coconut milk and 1/4 cup erythritol in a saucepan. Wait for it to boil and simmer for about one minute until the mix is slightly thick.
6. When the bread is done, remove it from the oven and cool it on a

baking rack.

7. Place the bread on a serving plate and drizzle with the caramel mixture.

8. Sprinkle the shredded coconut over the bread as well and then slice and serve!

Delicious Cheesecake

Servings Provided: 12

Prep & Cook Time: 52 minutes

Caloric Ratio Measure - Per Serving:

- Kcals: 231.8
- Net Carbohydrates: 3.4 g
- Protein: 4.9 g
- Fat Content: 22.3 g

Ingredients:

- Eggs (2)
- Sour cream (1.5 cups)
- Vanilla extract (2 tsp.)
- Keto-friendly granule sweetener - divided (.5 cup)
- Unchilled cream cheese (16 oz./450 g)
- Melted butter (2 tbsp.)
- Also Needed: 12 ramekins or 10-inch/25-cm springform pan

Preparation Technique:

1. Warm the oven temperature at 350° Fahrenheit/177° Celsius.
2. Whisk the eggs with the sour cream, vanilla, and sweetener in a big mixing container. Work in the cream cheese and butter.
3. Spoon and combine about ½ cup of the mixture into another bowl and add the raspberry flavoring.
4. Spoon the rest of the mix into the chosen container.
5. Scoop a portion of raspberry batter on top - swirl through the plain mixture.
6. Make a crust from ground almonds (1.5 cups), sweetener (.25 cup), and butter (.25 cup). Mix as a graham cracker crust - line the pan or ramekins.
7. Arrange the ramekins in a water bath or place a shallow pan with water in the oven below the ramekins/pan.
8. Bake for 20-25 minutes for ramekins or 35-40 minutes in a springform pan. The cake will firm up when refrigerated.
9. Top it off using fresh raspberries and whipped cream (not listed in the nutritional counts). Freeze if desired.

10.   *Note*: The nutritional calculations do not include crust.

Gingerbread Spice Dutch Baby

Servings Provided: 6

Prep & Cook Time: 30 minutes

Caloric Ratio Measure - Per Serving:

- Kcals: 256
- Net Carbohydrates: 2 g
- Fat Content: 24 g
- Protein: 8 g

Ingredients:

- Fresh unchilled heavy whipping cream/see recipe ch.1 (.75 cup)
- Unchilled eggs (5 large)
- Unchilled cream cheese - softened (2 oz./4 tbsp)
- Vanilla extract (1 tsp.)
- Maple extract (.5 tsp.)
- Powdered erythritol (.33 cup/1.5 oz./42 g)
- Unflavored whey protein isolate (2 tbsp.)
- Baking powder (1 tsp.)
- Salt (.25 tsp.)
- Ground ginger (1 tsp.)
- Ground cinnamon (.5 tsp.)
- Ground cloves (.25 tsp.)
- For the Pan: Unsalted butter (1.5 oz./3 tbsp./42 g)

- Ground cinnamon
- Powdered erythritol - for dusting
- Heavy whipping cream/see recipe ch.1
- Suggested: 10-inch/25 cm oven-proof skillet

Preparation Technique:

1. Set the oven setting to 400° Fahrenheit/204° Celsius.
2. Toss all of the fixings into a blender, except for the butter, blending till it's smooth and creamy. Blend for at least a minute to aerate the mixture. Set aside.
3. Add butter to the skillet and pop it into the oven. Once it's sizzling, transfer the pan to a cool spot and add the batter into the

center of the hot skillet.

4. Bake till the Dutch baby is puffy and browned (12-15 min.). The center should be just set.

5. Serve hot or cold with a dash of cinnamon, sprinkle of powdered sweetener, or a portion of freshly whipped cream.

Pumpkin Pie Cupcakes

Servings Provided: 6
Prep & Cook Time: 45 minutes
Caloric Ratio Measure - Per Serving:

- Kcals: 70
- Net Carbohydrates: 2.9 g
- Fat Content: 4.1 g
- Protein Count: 1.7 g

Ingredients:

- Coconut flour (3 tbsp.)
- Baking powder (.25 tsp.)
- Pumpkin pie spice (1 tsp.)
- Salt (1 pinch)
- Bak. soda (.25 tsp.)
- Egg (1 large)
- Pumpkin puree (.75 cup)
- Keto-friendly granular brown sugar (.33 cup)
- Heavy whipping cream/see recipe ch.1 (.25 cup)
- Vanilla (.5 tsp.)

Preparation Technique:

1. Warm up the oven to 350° Fahrenheit/177° Celsius.
2. Prepare the baking pan.
3. Sift the baking powder and soda with the salt and pumpkin pie spice.
4. In another container, mix the pumpkin puree with the cream, sweetener, vanilla, and egg until thoroughly incorporated.
5. Mix in the dry fixings. If the batter is too thin, whisk in an additional tablespoon of the coconut flour.
6. Portion into the muffin tins.
7. Bake until just puffed and barely set (25 to 30 min.).
8. Transfer the pan to the countertop (in the pan) to cool.
9. Store in the fridge for a minimum of one hour before it's time to serve.
10. Top it off using a generous helping of whipped

cream.

11.   Note: They will sink when you let them cook. It will be that much tastier with the serving of whipped cream!

Anytime Smoothies

Cinnamon Roll Smoothie

Servings Provided: 1
Prep & Cook Time: 5 minutes
Caloric Ratio Measure - Per Serving:
- Kcals: 145
- Net Carbohydrates: 0.6 g
- Fat Content: 3.3 g
- Protein: 26.5 g

Ingredients:
- Vanilla protein powder (2 tbsp.)
- Flax meal (1 tsp.)
- Almond milk (1 cup)
- Vanilla extract (.25 tsp.)
- Sweetener (4 tsp.)
- Cinnamon (.5 tsp.)
- Ice (1 cup)

Preparation Technique:

1. Toss the fixings into the blender.
2. Add ice and mix till it's creamy as desired.

Green Smoothie Delight

Servings Provided: 6 @ 1 cup each

Prep & Cook Time: 5 minutes **Caloric Ratio Measure - Per Serving**:

- Kcals: 37
- Net Carbohydrates: 3 g
- Fat Content: 4 g
- Protein: 1 g

Ingredients:

- Romaine lettuce (1 cup)
- Fresh chopped pineapple (.33 or 1/3 cup)
- Filtered water (4 cups)
- Fresh parsley (2 tbsp.)
- Fresh ginger (1 tbsp.)
- Kiwi fruit (.5 cup)
- Raw cucumber (1 cup)
- Avocado (half of 1)
- Granulated sugar substitute - swerve (1 tbsp.)

Preparation Technique:

1. Blend all of the ingredients until smooth.
2. Enjoy the leftovers for several days in the refrigerator.

Single-Serve Smoothie in a Bowl

Servings Provided: 1

Caloric Ratio Measure - Per Serving:
- Kcals: 570
- Net Carbohydrates: 4 grams
- Total Fat: 35 grams
- Protein: 35 grams

Ingredients Needed:
- Almond milk (.5 cup)
- Spinach (1 cup)
- Heavy cream (2 tbsp.)
- Low-carb protein powder (1 scoop)
- Coconut oil (1 tbsp.)
- Ice (2 cubes)

- Walnuts (4)
- Raspberries (4)
- Chia seeds (1 tsp.)
- Shredded coconut (1 tbsp.)

Preparation Steps:

1. Add a cup of spinach to your high-speed blender. Pour in the cream, almond milk, ice, and coconut oil.
2. Blend for a few seconds until it has an even consistency and all ingredients are well combined. Empty the goodies into a serving dish.
3. Arrange your toppings or give them a toss. Of course, you can make it pretty and alternate the strips of toppings.

Fat Bombs

Carrot Cake Fat Bombs

Servings Provided: 45 bombs

Prep & Cook Time: 1 hour 15 minutes

Caloric Ratio Measure - Per Serving:

- Kcals: 80.27
- Net Carbohydrates: 0.86 g
- Protein: 1.12 g
- Fat Content: 8.04 g

Ingredients:

- Grated carrots (.75 cup/100 g)
- Melted coconut manna (1 cup/224 g)
- Unchilled - salted butter (.5 cup/114 g)
- Unchilled cream cheese (.5 cup/114 g)
- Flax meal (2 tbsp./28 g)
- Chopped walnuts (1 cup/117 g)
- Cinnamon (2 tsp./5 g)
- Optional: Liquid keto-friendly sweetener (1 packet/as desired)

Preparation Technique:

1. Grate and add the carrots, coconut manna, cream cheese, butter, sweetener (if using), and flax meal in a food processor. Pulse until the fixings are thoroughly combined.
2. If the mixture is too soft to roll into balls, pop it into the fridge until you can easily handle it.
3. Meanwhile, prepare a baking tray with a layer of waxed or parchment baking paper. Roll the dough batch into (45) one-inch balls and place them in a single layer in the pan.
4. Sprinkle them using walnuts and cinnamon. Using the edges of the paper, toss until they are evenly coated. Gently press the coating into the bites and store the finished fat bombs in an airtight container in the refrigerator.

Pumpkin Spice Fat Bombs

Servings Provided: 24

Prep & Cook Time: 16 minutes

Caloric Ratio Measure - Per Serving:

- Kcals: 66
- Net Carbohydrates: 0.5 g
- Fat Content: 7 g
- Protein: 0.4 g

Ingredients:

- Unchilled butter (.5 cup/114 g)
- Unsweetened pumpkin puree (.25 cup/60 g)
- Coconut butter - melted but not hot (.5 cup/114 g)
- Cinnamon/combination of spices - ex. - cloves, allspice, nutmeg, etc. (1 tsp./3 g)

Preparation Technique:

1. Toss all of the fixings into a mixing container and mix until smooth.
2. Scoop the batter into silicone molds and taping them gently to remove air bubbles.
3. Freeze and enjoy once they are solid.

Strawberry Ginger Fat Bomb

Servings Provided: 28
Prep & Cook Time: 30 minutes
Caloric Ratio Measure - Per Serving:
- Kcals: 97
- Net Carbohydrates: 0.8 g
- Fat Content: 10 g
- Protein: 0.7 g

Ingredients:
- Coconut oil (4.2 oz./120 g)
- Coconut manna (120 g)
- Macadamia nuts - dry roasted with salt (120 g)
- Fresh ginger (0.4 oz./10 g)
- Fresh strawberries (120 g)
- Black pepper (1 pinch)

Preparation Technique:

1. Melt the coconut manna and oil in a glass bowl. (Use an electric mug warmer if you have one.)
2. Toss all of the fixings into a food processor fitted with a chopping blade. Puree until smooth.
3. Enjoy it - as is or freeze in a silicone mold so that the fat bombs will last much longer.

Appetizers

Bacon & Cheese Balls

Servings Provided: 4

Prep & Cook Time: 25 minutes

Caloric Ratio Measure - Per Serving:
- Kcals: 538
- Net Carbohydrates: 0.5 g
- Fat Content: 50 g
- Protein: 22 g

Ingredients:
- Cream cheese (6 oz. or 170 g)
- Sliced bacon (7 crumbled pieces)
- Gruyere shredded cheese (6 oz.)
- Unchilled butter (2 tbsp.)
- Red chili flakes (.5 tsp.)

Preparation Technique:

1. Fry the bacon in a skillet using the medium-temperature setting until it's crispy (5 min.).
2. Pour the grease into a bowl and combine it with the rest of the fixings (chili flakes, butter, cream, and gruyere cheese). Pop it into the fridge to set (15 min.).
3. Remove the mixture and mold it into small walnut-sized balls, and roll in the crumbled bacon to serve.

Crunchy Jalapeño Poppers

Servings Provided: 24
Prep & Cook Time: 45 minutes
Caloric Ratio Measure - Per Serving:
- Kcals: 98
- Net Carbohydrates: 1 g
- Protein: 4 g
- Fat Content: 8.5 g

Ingredients:
- Fresh jalapeño peppers (12-15/400 g)
- Unchilled cream cheese (8 oz. pkg./226 g)
- Shredded cheddar cheese (1 cup/112 g)
- Unchilled butter (4 tbsp./56 g)
- Cooked bacon (5 slices/45g)
- Pork rinds - crushed (1.75 oz. bag/50 g)
- The Topping: Cheddar cheese (.25 cup/28g)

Preparation Technique:

1. Warm the oven at 475° Fahrenheit/246° Celsius and cover a baking tray using a foil sheet.
2. Slice the peppers in half and remove the seeds. Add them onto the baking sheet cut side up.
3. Use an electric mixer to combine the cream cheese with the bacon crumbles, cheddar cheese, and butter in a mixing container.
4. Fill each pepper with the cheese filling. You can also add the filling to a plastic baggie. Remove the air, close, and snip one of the corners to add the filling.
5. Toss the crushed pork rinds into a mixing container. Gently push the cheese side of each pepper into the mixture to cover. Sprinkle a tiny bit of cheddar cheese over each one.
6. Bake the peppers in the upper third of the oven (10 min.). Adjust the oven setting to broil. Cook until the cheese has melted and browned.

Deli Roll-Ups

Servings Provided: 1

Prep & Cook Time: 6 minutes

Caloric Ratio Measure - Per Serving:

- Net Carbohydrates: 2 g
- Fat Content: 30 g
- Protein: 6 g

Ingredients:

- Iceberg lettuce - 1 whole leaf - flexible outer leaf (0.7 oz./21 g)
- Genoa salami - organic (0.6 oz./17 g)
- Creamy Italian Garlic Salad Dressing (0.6 oz./18 g)
- Mild-flavor keto-friendly oil of choice (0.5 oz./14 g)

Preparation Technique:

1. Use the leaf of one outer leaf of lettuce. (Do not use the hard-core stem.)
2. Place the salami in the leaf of lettuce. Fold in the edges, so it is the same width as the salami, and roll it. Tightly close the wrap using a toothpick.
3. Whisk the salad dressing and oil as a dip to serve.
4. Notes: The salad dressing and oil will separate as it sits. All you need to do is stir it again to combine.

Mini Eggplant Pizza

Servings Provided: 4

Prep & Cook Time: 17 minutes

Caloric Ratio Measure - Per Serving:
- Kcals: 119.1
- Net Carbohydrates: 5.7 g
- Fat Content: 7.5 g
- Protein: 4.9 g

Ingredients:
- Eggplant (1 @ 3 inches/8-cm - in diameter)
- Olive oil (4 tsp.)
- Salt (.5 tsp.)
- Black pepper (.125 tsp.)
- Pasta sauce (.25 cup)
- Mozzarella cheese - part-skim (.5 cup - shredded)

Preparation Technique:

1. Warm the oven or toaster oven at 425° Fahrenheit/218° Celsius.
2. Peel and slice both halves into four ½-inch slices.
3. Lightly brush all sides of the eggplant with oil and sprinkle using black pepper and salt.
4. Place them onto a baking tray to bake until browned and almost tender, turning once (6-8 min.).
5. Spread one tablespoon of pasta sauce over each eggplant slice with a sprinkle of shredded cheese.
6. Bake until the cheese melts (3-5 min.). Serve hot.

Naruto Rolls

Servings Provided: 3
Prep & Cook Time: 30 minutes
Caloric Ratio Measure - Per Serving:

- Kcals: 81
- Net Carbohydrates: 2 g
- Fat Content: 5 g
- Protein: 7 g

Ingredients:

- Cucumber (1 long)
- Avocado (half of 1)
- Raw salmon (3 slices)

Preparation Technique:

1. Remove the peel and slice the cucumber using a vegetable slicer.
2. Line the sushi roll on a cutting block with a layer of cling film under it.
3. Place the cucumber slices vertically, overlapping each one.
4. Slice the avocado and place it horizontally over the cucumber slices, and add the slices of salmon.
5. Roll it and gently press the ends to wrap it with a cling film to hold its shape.
6. Pop it into the freezer to set (10-15 min.).
7. Discard the plastic wrap and slice to serve.

Sweet Mustard Mini Sausages

Servings Provided: 4

Prep & Cook Time: 20 minutes

Caloric Ratio Measure- Per Serving:
- Kcals: 744
- Net Carbohydrates: 7.2 g
- Protein: 24 g
- Fat Content: 45 g

Ingredients:
- Keto-friendly brown sugar - ex. Swerve (1 cup)
- Mustard powder (2 tsp.)
- Almond flour (3 tbsp.)
- White vinegar (.25 cup)
- Lemon juice (.25 cup)
- Tamari sauce (1 tsp.)
- Mini smoked sausages (2 lb./910 g)

Preparation Technique:

1. Whisk the mustard with the sugar substitute and flour in a saucepan. Mix in tamari sauce, vinegar, and juice.
2. Set the burner using the medium temperature setting. Once boiling, stir about two minutes until thickened.
3. Mix in the sausages and gently stir to cook for about five minutes.
4. Serve the delicious treat at any time.

Zucchini Nacho Chips

Servings Provided: 4
Prep & Cook Time: 35 minutes
Caloric Ratio Measure - Per Serving:

- Kcals: 66
- Net Carbohydrates: 1.6 g
- Fat Content: 6.9 g
- Protein: 0.6 g

Ingredients:

- Zucchini (1 large)
- Taco seasoning (1 tbsp.)
- Coconut oil (to fry)
- Salt (as needed)

Preparation Technique:

1. Use a mandolin to slice the zucchini. Place them over the sink in a colander and drizzle with salt. Wait five minutes and press out the water.
2. Prepare a pan or skillet (350° Fahrenheit/177° Celsius) to heat the oil.
3. Add the zucchini (working in batches) or about 20 chips at a time.
4. Drain the grease on a paper towel-lined platter and serve with a sprinkle of the taco seasoning of choice.

Snacks

Cheesecake Mocha Bars

Servings Provided: 16
Prep & Cook Time: 45-50 minutes
Caloric Ratio Measure - Per Serving:
- Kcals: 232
- Net Carbohydrates: 3.2 g
- Fat Content: 21 g
- Protein: 6 g

Ingredients:

The Brownie Layer:
- Vanilla extract (2 tsp.)
- Unsalted butter (6 tbsp.)
- Large eggs (3)
- Almond flour (1.5 cups)
- Baking cocoa - your favorite (.5 cup)
- Erythritol (1 cup)
- Salt (.5 tsp.)
- Instant coffee (.5 tbsp.)
- Baking powder (1 tsp.)

- Large egg (1)
- Softened cream cheese (1 lb. or 450 g)
- Erythritol (.5 cup)
- Vanilla extract (1 tsp.)
- Also Needed: 20x20-cm/8x8-inch baking pan

Preparation Technique:

1. Set the oven temperature to 350° Fahrenheit/177° Celsius.
2. Lightly grease or spray the pan.
3. Combine the wet fixings starting with the butter and vanilla. Next, fold in the eggs.
4. Use another container to combine the dry fixings and whisk with the wet fixings. Set aside ¼ of a cup of the batter for later. Pour

the mixture into the pan.

5. Mix the cream cheese (room temperature) with the rest of the ingredients for the second layer. Spread it on the sheet of brownies.

6. Use the reserved batter as the last layer (will be thin). Bake the bars for 30 to 35 minutes.

7. When it's cooled, slice the cheesecake bars, and serve.

Chocolate Loaf Bread

Servings Provided: 16

Prep & Cook Time: 1 hour 10 minutes

Caloric Ratio Measure - Per Serving:
- Kcals: 115.2
- Net Carbohydrates: 1.5 g
- Fat Content: 9.5 g
- Protein: 4.3 g

Ingredients:
- Baking powder (2 tsp.)
- Almond flour (1 cup)
- Sea salt (.25 tsp.)
- Organic ground flax seeds (3 tbsp.)
- 100% Cocoa - special dark (4 tbsp.)
- Keto-friendly sugar replacement - ex. swerve-type (1 cup)
- Egg (6 large)
- Olive oil (4 tbsp.)
- Vanilla extract (1 tsp.)

Preparation Technique:

1. Warm the oven to 350° Fahrenheit/177° Celsius.
2. Spray a loaf pan with a spritz of cooking oil spray. Mix the almond flour with the ground flax seeds, baking powder, dark cocoa powder, sea salt, and confectioner's sugar in a food processor. Blitz until smooth.
3. Mix in the eggs, oil, and vanilla extract. Pulse until smooth.
4. Dump it into the pan. Set a timer and bake until the loaf center is cooked through (45-50 min.).
5. Cool for 20 minutes before running a butter knife around the loaf edges and unmolding the loaf.
6. Slice into 16 portions and top with your favorite fruits.

Chocolate & Orange Chunk Cookies

Servings Provided: 16

Prep & Cook Time: 35 minutes

Caloric Ratio Measure - Per Serving:

- Kcals: 159.1
- Net Carbohydrates: 2.3 g
- Fat Content: 14.5 g
- Protein: 4.37 g

Ingredients:

- Butter (7 tbsp.)
- Almond flour (2 cups)
- Granulated sweetener (.75 cup)
- Dark chocolate (2 oz./56 g)
- Eggs (2 large)
- Orange zest (1 tbsp.)
- Vanilla extract (1 tsp.)
- Orange extract (1 tsp.)
- Orange juice (1 tbsp.)
- Bak. powder (.75 tsp.)
- Salt (.5 tsp.)
- Bak. soda (.5 tsp.)

Preparation Technique:

1. Set the oven temperature at 350° Fahrenheit/177° Celsius.
2. Combine the dry fixings (baking soda, salt, flour, baking powder, and sweetener) in a large mixing bowl.
3. Using a microwavable dish, melt the butter and stir in the orange extract, orange zest, juice, and vanilla extract. Combine all of the fixings, mixing well.
4. Add the dough onto a baking tin, shaping it into a rectangle. Slice it into 16 servings. Bake for 20 to 22 minutes. Cool for about ten minutes, and enjoy it.

Chocolate Sea Salt Cookies

Servings Provided: 15
Prep & Cook Time: 30 minutes
Caloric Ratio Measure - Per Serving:
- Kcals: 188
- Net Carbohydrates: 1.6 g
- Fat Content: 18.2 g
- Protein: 3.5 g

Ingredients:
- Unchilled coconut oil (.75 cup)
- Eggs (2)
- Vanilla extract (1 tsp.)
- Keto-friendly - golden monk fruit sweetener (.75 cup)
- Unsweetened cocoa powder (2 tbsp.)
- Salt (.5 tsp.)
- Cream of tartar (.25 tsp.)
- Baking soda (.5 tsp.)
- Almond flour (2 cups)
- Flaky sea salt (as desired)

Preparation Technique:

1. Set the oven temperature to reach 350° Fahrenheit/177° Celsius.
2. Set up two baking sheets with a layer of parchment baking paper.
3. Prepare using a hand mixer. Combine the eggs, coconut oil, and vanilla extract in a large bowl.
4. Toss in the sweetener, baking soda, cocoa powder, salt, and cream of tartar. Mix thoroughly.
5. Gradually fold in the almond flour. Form the dough into balls. Place onto the baking sheet. Arrange them about two to three inches apart.
6. Garnish using the sea salt on top of each cookie.
7. Bake cookies for about 16 to 20 minutes - baking one tray at a time.
8. Remove and cool completely.
9. Gently pull the paper away from each of the cookies to serve.

Sunflower Seed Surprise Cookies

Servings Provided: 12
Prep & Cook Time: 20 minutes
Caloric Ratio Measure - Per Serving:
- Kcals: 69
- Net Carbohydrates: 0.64 g
- Protein: 2.3 g
- Fat Content: 6.3 g

Ingredients:
- Egg (50 g/1 large egg)
- Sugar-free sunflower seed butter (.75 cup/100 g)
- Coconut oil (16 g/1 rounded tbsp.)
- Vanilla extract (2 g/.5 tsp.)
- Salt - Baking powder & soda (1 g/1 pinch each)

Preparation Technique:

1. Warm the oven temperature setting to 350° Fahrenheit/177° Celsius.
2. Set the rack in the upper portion of the oven.
3. Prepare a cookie tray using a layer of parchment baking paper.
4. Mix all of the fixings in a large container.
5. Roll and flatten the mixture into 12 balls about the width of a quarter.
6. Bake the cookies for seven to nine minutes until they're firm in the center.
7. Cool the cookies for a couple of hours.

Conclusion

I hope you have enjoyed each section of your new book, *3 Weeks of Ketogenic Recipes.* I hope it was informative and provided you with all of the tools you need to achieve your goals - whatever they may be. The next step is to gather a shopping list and head to your marketplace!

These are a few more recommendations that might help if you want to dine out with keto:

- *Breakfast Suggestions:* Sometimes, there is nothing better than eggs if you want to play it safe. You may be off on some of the counts, but after some practice, you will know how to gauge your eating habits for the most important meal of the day.

- *Lunchtime Suggestions:* Chicken and fish are usually good choices. Many restaurants now offer diet-friendly menus. Select a chicken salad or a regular salad. Just be cautious of the dressing used. Try some vinaigrette or plain vinegar.

- *Dinner Suggestions:* Always choose a fresh green veggie with a lean cut of meat as your main course. Try something in the hamburger line minus the bun or a tempting entrée of broccoli and steak.

Have some fun and reap the benefits!

Finally, if you found this book useful in any way, a review on Amazon is always appreciated!